Praise for *Sports Hypnosis in*

CW00765865

As an experienced hypnotherapist and
ing and gaining from well written, struc̲t̲u̲r̲e̲d̲ ̲b̲o̲o̲k̲s̲ ̲o̲n̲ ̲h̲y̲p̲n̲o̲s̲i̲s̲,
and I have read many! I like nothing more than to peruse people's
views, ideas, and practice to expand and enhance my own. This book
was one of those pleasurable reads taking me through the author's
views, strategies, techniques, and case studies on hypnosis in sports
performance.

It is clear from the skilful writing that experience and personal successes are the foundations to each chapter, thus it is a fascinating read
not just for all those interested in finely tuning their existing hypnotic
interventions, but for anyone involved in sports performance or
simply interested in this field.

This book's strength is not just the knowledge it delivers, but its comprehensive structure and readability. It is a first rate example of multi-
level communication conveyed through the written word.

It is packed full of motivational ideas including metaphors and stories, scripts, strategies, and suggestions all entwined around real
sports performers, which will undoubtedly leave you energized about
the efficiency and effectiveness of sports hypnosis.

Well done Joseph!

**Tom Barber, DHp MA, Director, Contemporary College of
Therapeutic Studies UK, co-author of *Thinking Therapeutically:
Hypnotic Skills and Strategies Explored***

An excellent read for sports psychologists, sports therapists and lov-
ers of sport. Techniques that work are all backed up by a wealth of
experience.

Aaron Surtees, Director, City Hypnosis

In this very practical book on hypnosis and sports, Joseph Tramontana
adds to his string of effective publications. His tone is approachable
and friendly. Clearly, he has a wide background in hypnosis, which
he makes accessible for the novice as well as the experienced clinician.

Joe's approach is straightforward: you don't need to be an accomplished athlete in order to be a good mental coach. The stories of his

clinical work and extensive contacts with sports luminaries make it easy for the reader to get involved. In addition to many scripts, he gives suggestions on how to talk to coaches and athletes in order to market a viable sport hypnosis practice.

David M. Wark, PhD, ABPH, Emeritus Professor of Psychology, University of Minnesota

The increasing popularity of mental training in sport, and in particular sports hypnosis, has created a need for a comprehensive practical guide for hypnotherapists and sports psychologists interested in developing their hypnosis skills in performance-related fields. In *Sports Hypnosis in Practice*, Joseph Tramontana has produced such a guide, filled with case studies, interviews, and scripts from his many years of experience as a clinical sports psychologist. The book details the methods he has used in a variety of sports, including the actual hypnosis scripts used in sessions, as well as providing considerable reference to the research and reading on which these methods are based.

Based on accepted sports psychology principles, *Sports Hypnosis in Practice* goes beyond just introducing hypnosis to sports psychology, but also examines the role of mental training as a whole, including insightful interviews with coaches and former players. In addition to chapters covering specific sports such as golf, tennis, athletics, and show jumping, Dr Tramontana has included useful guidance for dealing with other issues such as injury recovery and substance abuse. For the experienced hypnotherapist wanting to expand into sport, or the sports psychologist wanting to learn about adding hypnosis to their skillset, this book is an invaluable addition to their library.

Gary Baker, The Centre for Sports Hypnosis

Anyone serious about hypnotic sport psychology will insist on having this book in their library. The chapters on working with the injured athlete returning to their sport and with the addicted athlete are both unique and most valuable. Taking the information in this book and individualizing and tailoring it to the sportsperson actually sitting in front of you will garner great results!

John H. Edgette, PsyD, Director of the Milton H. Erickson Institute of Philadelphia, and co-author of *Winning the Mind Game*

Hypnotherapists who enjoy working with athletes or who want to add sports psychology to their practice will cheer for Joseph Tramontana's *Sports Hypnosis in Practice*. Unlike other fine books that address hypnosis for a specific sport (like Tom Saunders' *Golf*) or a generic approach to hypnosis for all sports (like Edgette and Rowan's *Winning the Mind Game*), this book devotes chapters to 15 individual and team sports – from gymnastics to rugby.

The book opens with an overview of the literature on sports hypnosis and the emergence of sports psychology. The first chapter gives information on general considerations for the practitioner, such as introducing sports hypnosis to the client, tests of hypnotizability, hypnotic inductions, deepening, guided imagery, self-hypnosis, regression, reframing, and cognitive behavioral therapy. The subsequent chapters, on hypnotic approaches to specific sports, show practitioners that each sport has its own vocabulary and performance standards. The author writes from his own experience as a runner and as a hypnotherapist who has worked with many athletes; amateurs and professionals.

Like Tramontana's *Hypnotically Enhanced Treatment for Addictions*, this book is highly readable with excellent case examples (many of which can be used as metaphors), hypnotic scripts, treatment strategies, and verbatim interviews with coaches and athletes about the psychology behind specific sports. A chapter on helping athletes recover from injury includes pain management, imagery for healing, and a hypnotic question–answer process for pinpointing the origin of psychosomatic illness. The final chapter on addictions and eating disorders in sports is as timely as today's sports headlines. This book hits a home run!

Judith E. Pearson, PhD, Professional Counselor, Clinical Hypnotherapist, Master NLP Practitioner/Trainer, and author of
The Weight, Hypnotherapy and You Weight Reduction Program: An NLP and Hypnotherapy Practitioner's Manual

Dr Tramontana has written a excellent book on the practice of sports hypnosis. This is a book that I can now highly recommend to my future students. He has cited the top people in the field of sports hypnosis and I am sure that all of them will be making this book required reading for anyone interested in using hypnosis with athletes.

Mitch Smith, LCSW-C, DAHB

Where were you Dr Tramontana when I needed you about 15 years ago? The telephone rang and, on answering, I heard a very cultured female voice telling me that she needed my help to improve her golf!

I needed patients but had to admit to her, in all honesty, that I hardly knew one end of a golf club from the other. If she was happy with that then I was prepared to do all that I could.

She came and for a couple of sessions we used the first half of the session for her to explain the mechanics of her need – the smooth swing and so on, and the second half introducing all of this hypnotically.

She was happy. I wasn't. As we progressed I broached the idea that her problem was more her own self-belief and confidence than any physical malfunction. Greater belief in her own abilities and a more relaxed outlook on her game would lead to its own steady improvement.

To begin with I think she was rather offended by me inferring that she was uptight, lacking in confidence, angry with herself, but was prepared to go along with me and let me drop the "golf coaching" and concentrate on what I knew best as a hypnotherapist.

The results were terrific. She went from strength to strength and in a short time started to feature regularly on the "roll of honour" at her club.

Other club members asked her what she was doing to bring about this improvement. Was she having private lessons? She did admit to visiting "her man in Tewkesbury." It was assumed I was a golf pro who had taken up coaching. They asked for my details as they wished to see the same improvement in their own games. My phone never rang though. As soon as they realized I was a hypnotherapist and not a golfer they rapidly lost interest and added: "We don't need that sort of man thank you!"

Times have changed – fortunately – and it is now commonplace to hear of sports psychologists and so on, working with our leading sportsmen and women. Joseph Tramontana's *Sports Hypnosis in Practice* is a groundbreaking book explaining how hypnosis can best be used to the benefit of those who are in sport and are seeking to achieve their peak performance.

In my own experience the client had in her mind that I could, through hypnosis, teach her how to play golf better. As Joseph Tramontana says in his book, this is not the task of the therapist but is the job of the coach. It is for them to develop and extend the mechanical side to boost physical performance.

The hypnotherapist, sports counselor or sports psychologist is there to work on all mental aspects of sport. Importantly, and a great relief to a sports illiterate such as myself, the therapist does not need to be familiar with the sport or the physical activity to be able to be effective and efficient in the role of "mental coach" to the sports people who come to him/her.

This fact is, indeed, one of the main focuses of the book. The author refers to his own experience and says: "I have had successful outcomes in working with athletes across many sports that I have never played."

The book is an excellent mix of strategies and scripts. We are given detailed outlines and in-depth explanations of how to work with a client, and the scripts are extensive and excellent. We are taught how to help the subject relax, concentrate, and become more focused so that they are more able to achieve maximum potential.

We see that the hypnosis road can lead the sportsperson to achieve a better balance in life. For so many the effort to succeed becomes a struggle between achieving physical prowess and improving skill and achievement, often at the risk of allowing mental fragility to threaten to wreck the path of progress. Many of the prima donnas we see on our football pitches would see their game improve if only they had more skill in managing their mental body. Hypnosis is an excellent medium for changing behavior, for improving focus, concentration, calm, anger management, and much more. Fear and lack of confidence or self-belief can also be enhanced. The coach can deal with the physical.

Put the two together and we stand the chance of producing the balanced sportsperson who is able to produce the goods in all areas.

The book is of great interest in that it gives a wide variety of case studies where the author has worked successfully with sportsperson during his career. Very insightful and fascinating. In particular I liked the fact that many of the sportsmen and women would talk to him, perhaps years down the line, and be able to recount in great detail their hypnotic experiences and techniques. The value was seen clearly and was very well received and, as a result, became part of the everyday tool bag of success for countless athletes. They acknowledge, without reservation, the enormous benefit it has brought them.

The author leaves no stone unturned. We hear constantly of sports injury and also, sadly, of drug abuse in sport. Both of these are given time and space within the book and we are offered insight and help into how best to assist an athlete returning from injury or addiction. Inspirational and very illuminating.

There is also a section on affirmations which I just loved:

"Life is 10 percent what happens to you, and 90 percent how you respond to it!"

"Put your heart, mind, intellect and soul even to your smallest acts. This is the secret of success."

"I don't know the key to success, but the key to failure is trying to please everybody."

When being given this book to review I thought, "Oh dear, sport!" I need not have worried.

This book is an excellent reference book and handbook for any therapist to dip into to find the tools, techniques, and strategies for success when dealing with clients who seek help in relation to their sporting life.

It is a book I am delighted to recommend and I feel that it has the potential of becoming a bestseller in this age where sport is so pressurised yet, a far cry from my early experience, where its participants are far more open minded and aware that so much of their success stems from their thoughts not just from their raw physical talent.

David Slater, BA, DHyp, MHA(RegHyp), MASC, DCS, MGSCT, Clinical Hypnotherapist and Counselor

Sports Hypnosis
in Practice

Sports Hypnosis in Practice

Scripts, Strategies, and Case Examples

Joseph Tramontana, PhD

Crown House Publishing Limited
www.crownhouse.co.uk
www.crownhousepublishing.com

First published by

Crown House Publishing Ltd
Crown Buildings, Bancyfelin, Carmarthen, Wales, SA33 5ND, UK
www.crownhouse.co.uk

and

Crown House Publishing Company LLC
6 Trowbridge Drive, Suite 5, Bethel, CT 06801-2858, USA
www.crownhousepublishing.com

© Joseph Tramontana 2011

The right of Joseph Tramontana to be identified as the author of this
work has been asserted by him in accordance with the Copyright,
Designs and Patents Act 1988.

All rights reserved. Except as permitted under current legislation no part of this
work may be photocopied, stored in a retrieval system, published, performed in
public, adapted, broadcast, transmitted, recorded or reproduced in any form or
by any means, without the prior permission of the copyright owners.
Enquiries should be addressed to
Crown House Publishing Limited.

British Library Cataloguing-in-Publication Data
A catalogue entry for this book is available
from the British Library.

ISBN 978-184590679-5
LCCN 2010937324

Printed and bound in the USA

This book is dedicated to my sister, Pamela, who is no longer with us, and my other three sisters, Emily, Susan, and Terri, all very special in their individual ways. All four sisters could run faster than any of the boys in the neighborhood, except for me, of course. Also, to my wife, Lynn; my children Jim and Jody; and step-children, Tori and Tre'; as well as my grandchildren, who are such a joy.

Acknowledgments

I wish to thank Brian Kinchen, former National Football League tight end and long snapper, whose story is told in a condensed form in Chapter 6 and coaches Tony Minnis (Louisiana State University (LSU) women's tennis coach), Yvette Girouard (LSU women's softball coach), and Leaf Boswell (coach of LSU's equestrian club team) for their openness and willingness to talk about the mental side of their sports. In addition, many thanks to the former athlete-clients who agreed to be interviewed for this book – golfers Greg Conley and Lizette Lee (Pietro) and volleyball player Paige Huber-Pitts – all with whom I so enjoyed working. There are many other athletes with whom I have worked who are not mentioned by name in the case examples for a variety of reasons; however, as well as teaching them about the mental side of sports, I feel I have learned from all of them.

Contents

Introduction

I like to postulate that some types of hypnosis or self-hypnosis must have been used back in the days of the Roman gladiators, or perhaps even earlier. How else could someone enter an arena with a lion and contemplate his impending demise without at least being able to disassociate to some extent? I also muse as to how in those days this activity was seen as "sport" in the eyes of the emperors and the viewing public, but a life-or-death experience by the gladiators themselves.

The psychology of sport is becoming an increasingly popular field of study and practice for psychologists. Two recent books are James Loehr's *The new toughness training for sports* (1995) which has a foreword by Chris Evert and Dan Jansen (Loehr has worked with many other famous athletes) and Jack Lesyk's *Developing sport psychology within your clinical practice* (1998) which includes a brief discussion on relaxation training (pp. 65–66), which he refers to as "a sort of light hypnosis." William Morgan has a chapter on hypnosis in sport and exercise psychology in Van Raalte and Brewer's *Exploring sport and exercise psychology* (2002).

I had the opportunity to chat with Dr Loehr following his Keynote Address at the Association of Applied Sports Psychology (AASP) Annual Conference in Providence (Loehr, 2010). As CEO and Chairman of the Human Performance Institute in Orlando, Florida, he works to enhance performance with corporations and military special forces, as well as athletes, but the techniques he employs are similar across all groups. He said he had moved away from using hypnosis as a technique with athletes because he did not want them to feel that he was the one in control of their improvement. He agreed, however, that my focus on training the athlete in self-hypnosis helped to negate that concern.

At the 2010 AASP conference there was not one presentation on hypnosis in sports in four days of lectures, symposia, and workshops, although I did hear a speaker make a perfunctory mention of hypnosis for relaxation. However, I found it interesting that this group – a cross-section of psychologists, sports counselors, exercise physiologists, educators, and so on – talked about many of the same techniques I use albeit without the use of formal hypnotic induction or self-hypnotic training. For example, they discussed relaxation, concentration, mindfulness, focus, centering, visualization, and a great deal about imagery. Many of the presentations dealt with mental skills training (they referred to it as MST), which to some extent incorporates these same techniques as well as others such as goal-setting.

At one of the social events, I met a sports counselor from New York. When I told him about this forthcoming book, he exclaimed: "You have scripts? I need them!" When I suggested he could wait a few months and buy the book, he responded: "I can't wait that long. I need them now!" This encounter served to reinforce my thesis that sports hypnosis is indeed a specialized form of sports psychology.

A number of university psychology departments now have specific training in Sports Psychology, and the American Psychological Association (APA) has a membership division (Division 47, Sports and Exercise Psychology). There is also the Association of Applied Sports Psychology, with over 1,500 members, and the National Institute of Sports Professionals (NISP), as well as other organizations for sports counselors. The *Journal of Applied Sport Psychology* caters to research in this area and Routledge/Psychology Press has a catalog of titles in the field, as does Human Kinetics, the latter describing itself as "the information leader in physical activity."

In a recent review by Schwartz in the APA's *Monitor on Psychology* (2008), she reports how psychologists are increasingly being called upon to help Olympians improve their concentration, focus their skills, and cope with the intense pressure of competition at such a high level. She reports the responses of 11 psychologists who are involved in this field. Margaret Ottley, for example, who works with the US Track and Field Team, reinforces those skills athletes already use, including breathing techniques, positive self-talk, and sensory awareness. Colleen Hacker says that with the US Field Hockey Team, she relies on performance-enhancement techniques such as imagery, focusing, distraction control, and pre-performance routines. She attempts to aid them in being their best more often and to play their best when it counts most. Other respondents in different events gave similar descriptions.

In an article from a recent American Society of Clinical Hypnosis (ASCH) newsletter titled "Report from the president's desk" (Fall 2008), Wark wrote about the First World Congress on Excellence in Sports and Life held in Beijing, China in August, 2008. He noted that the conference brought together mental trainers from sports, business coaching, education, and health, all of whom were interested in the application of hypnosis as an aspect of mental training. All of this is noted to point out the increasing popularity in the field.

Experts from various theoretical backgrounds talk about the significance of our beliefs and the mental models or mindsets that shape our behavior (see Bandler & Grinder, 1979; Dyer, 2004; Ellis & Harper, 1975; Meichenbaum, 1977). It is generally accepted that we act and perform in accordance with the beliefs our minds tell us are true. Many of the affirmations presented on pages 153 to 160 suggest that if you think something is not possible or out of reach, you're probably not going to invest much energy toward attaining that goal. To unlearn old self-doubts, we must substitute new, more productive thinking. The management by objectives approach employed in industry suggests the following three steps:

1. Identify the specific goals or results you desire to achieve.
2. Then create and develop actions (objectives) that will accomplish those results.
3. Determine the methods (steps) necessary to achieve these objectives.

So if you want to achieve your goals, you must create a mindset consistent with beliefs that support the truth you want in your future (hypnotherapists refer to this as "future projection" or "age progression").

As will be shown in this book, it is important for the hypnosis practitioner to be familiar with the basic tenets of sports psychology so that he or she can adapt these strategies to hypnotic presentation. I have been using hypnosis and hypnotherapy since 1978 for a wide variety of applications including smoking cessation, weight loss therapy, and other addictions such as alcoholism and problem drinking, drug abuse/addictions, and pathological gambling (Tramontana, 2008a, 2009a). I have also used hypnosis for pain control during surgical procedures (Tramontana, 2008b), as well as many other areas in which I have not published, including lowering subjective pain with chronic pain patients, decreasing anxiety, obsessive-compulsive behaviors, fear of public speaking, trichotil-lomania, bedwetting, improving study habits and exam taking.

While there are some studies that specifically address sports hypnosis in the literature, there is not much on the efficacy of the hypnotic approach. Books that explicitly address sports hypnosis include *Golf: Lower your score with mental training* by Tom Saunders (2005), which refers primarily to mental training but has sections on hypnosis and self-hypnosis training, John Edgette and Tim Rowan's *Winning the mind game* (2003), and Donald Liggett's *Sport hypnosis* (2000).

Furthermore, while a wide range of generic scripts have been published, there is a dearth of scripts for working with athletes in their specific sports. The generic ones include a script in Allen (2004, pp. 325–327) that focuses on sports performance in general, while Havens and Walters (1989) provide scripts for maximizing performance (pp. 141, 161). In Hammond's (1990) book of scripts, which functions as a cookbook for beginning hypnotherapists, there is a brief focus on arousal level and sports performance (pp. 466–467). Pratt and Korn (1996, p. 337) respond to questions regarding the efficacy of hypnosis in enhancing sports perform-ance by providing some basic information on how it might apply. They include an example of how Ken Norton used self-hypnosis to prepare for the bout in which he beat Mohammad Ali. They note that he was already a very good boxer, so this technique did not suddenly transform him into a winner; rather, it helped him perform at his best.

Some authors suggest that therapists should only work with ath-letes in sports in which they have personal experience of playing. As will be seen in my approach, I disagree with this theory. While I have had experience of playing football, running track (sprints) and distance running, including five years coaching marathon run-ners, as well as having played basketball, baseball, and soccer as an adolescent, my belief is that the therapist need not have played the sport to be effective in what I refer to as *hypnotic coaching*. I have had successful outcomes in working with athletes across many sports that I have never played.

One of my early experiences in the application of hypnosis, shortly after attending a sports hypnosis workshop (Pulos and Smith,

1998), was with a female high school high jumper. I instructed the girl's mother to ask her coach to write down for me some of the key phrases she attempted to instill in her high jumpers and I reinforced these hypnotically, with rapid and dramatic success. This case is presented in Chapter 3. This general approach can be seen in many of the chapters in terms of how I determined a course of hypnotic suggestion when dealing with sports in which I had no personal experience.

There are many more books on sports psychology, and I see sports hypnosis as a sub-specialty of sports psychology. Especially prevalent are publications on golf such as Timothy Gallwey's *The inner game of golf* (1981), Tom Saunders' *Golf: Lower your score through mental training* (2005), and three books by Robert Rotella: *Golf is not a game of perfect* (1995), *Golf is a game of confidence* (1996), and *The golfer's mind* (2004), to name but a few. Gallwey had previously published *The inner game of tennis* (1974) and *Inner skiing* (1977), and in 1997 revised both. He demonstrates how the mental aspects of a sport generalize across many sports. He notes that ever since he missed a heartbreakingly easy volley on match point in the National Junior Tennis Championships at the age of 15, he has been fascinated with the problem of how humans interfere with their own ability to achieve and learn.

I have found these books and studies invaluable as a starting point to understanding the specific needs that plug into enhanced performance in a variety of sports. In my practice, I give clients some of the same suggestions that are offered conversationally by sports psychologists – albeit I deliver them when the client is in a hypnotic state.

In general, most sports psychologists focus on cognitive behavioral approaches to teach athletes effective thinking – the use of positive thoughts during competition. Much of the literature on cognitive behavioral therapy (CBT) originated with Ellis and Harper (1975) and Meichenbaum (1977). In essence, modifying either cognition (thinking) or behavior should modify the other. The primary focus, however, has been on changing the behaviors by altering thinking/cognition. I believe that hypnosis is an excellent example of how behavior can be changed first, through hypnotic intervention, and the resultant shift in thinking follows. An example is a client who describes a fear of public speaking. A strict cognitive approach would be to attempt to alter the individual's behaviors by changing his or her thinking about public speaking. My experience, however, is that by using hypnotic techniques to help clients feel relaxed and calm while giving a talk, their subsequent thinking about their effectiveness as a public speaker becomes much more positive and the fear or anxiety dissipates.

Williams and Leffingwell (2002, pp. 75–76) write about how athletic performance is affected by what athletes think about themselves, their situation, and performance – and how this then impacts on their feelings and behavior. Pulos (1990) describes how high performance individuals know the power of self-talk. They have a system for programming themselves with positive messages which feed their cycle of self-esteem and self-confidence. He notes that positive self-talk emphasizes what can be done, not what might go wrong. He adds that negative self-chatter drains energy and creates toxic effects within individuals, while positive self-talk can create a psychic fountain which nourishes all aspects of one's being. He describes self-talk as nothing more than "everyday waking hypnosis."

While some sporting competition happens so fast that there isn't much time to think during the event (e.g., a 100 meter sprint), others allow space for a great deal of self-talk, especially endurance sports. Even those sports that are fast-paced, however, allow for frequent negative self-talk, as will be seen in Chapter 3 on running and Chapter 8 on tennis.

I like to use stories and anecdotes about great athletes with clients to demonstrate the importance of the mental aspect of their games. In an article titled "Mental edge," Hodenfield (2009) refers to the fact that winning takes more than muscles, strategy, and execution, stating: "The ability to win often comes down to sheer, ice-cold nerve." He refers to a number of world-class athletes at the top of their games such as tennis star Serena Williams, golf's Tiger Woods, skateboarding idol Tony Hawk, skier Lindsey Vonn, NASCAR driver Brian Vickers, and past football great John Elway. He quotes Serena Williams as saying: "You have to have the desire to achieve, to do better and do more and continually do, do, do. It's an insatiable desire to not only win, but not to lose." On Tiger Woods, he notes: "Very little in Tiger Woods' physical motions resemble those of his childhood hero, Jack Nicklaus. The one tool they share is their most lethal weapon: An unshakeable, unwavering ability to concentrate." He adds that John Elway's business adviser stated: "That ability to think quickly and process is what he used in his playing days when he read defenses quickly. That's probably why he was the greatest ever at the two-minute drill."

Billie Jean King is one of the greatest players in tennis history. In addition to being a famous female champion, she is widely known for her cross-gender match with Bobby Riggs which many say opened the door for equal treatment of women in sports. Her book, *Pressure is a privilege* (2008) describes seeing pressure as a positive or "opportunistic emotion" which produces energy and makes it easier to focus and concentrate on what is happening now.

There are several reasons why I consider sports hypnosis to be an attractive sub-specialty of hypnosis or psychotherapy practice. First, I find it to be a fun and exciting sub-area of my general psychological practice. Typically athletes are not coming to see me because of psychological disturbance; rather they are seeking self-improvement in their sport. Second, the progress, gains, and successes are often quick, dramatic, and measurable. Third, since there isn't a diagnosable mental condition, and treatment is not reimbursable by insurance companies, it is strictly on a private-pay basis. Finally, athletes are highly motivated to improve and are used to repetition in practicing their sport, so they are usually equally accepting of the need to practice self-hypnosis.

Occasionally, a client who has had a fall or other injury will present with a fear or anxiety about competing, and this can be handled well through hypnotherapy. For example, the athlete may be desensitized in much the same manner as a phobic patient would be. With one professional golfer with whom I worked, there was a psychological reason why he kept barely failing to "make the cut" (this case is discussed in Chapter 2). Because golf is so popular internationally and across many ability levels, I have had more requests for hypnosis from golfers than for any other sport. There appear to be many more participants, both amateur and professional, seeking any methods available to improve their golf scores. Consequently, Chapter 2 is the longest.

In the following chapters, strategies, scripts, and case examples will be presented in a number of sports for athletes with whom I have personally worked who desired to improve their perform-ance. The sports covered include track and field (runners and jumpers); gymnasts and cheerleaders; equestrian competition; baseball, basketball, and football (the US "big three"); softball; ten-nis; volleyball; soccer; and Olympic shooting.

One interesting phenomenon described in Chapter 5 in working with equestrian show jumpers is the principle of everything "slow-ing down." This "slow motion" phenomenon is similar to what I believe happens in other sports, although it is often just written off as "experience." For example, the better professional football quarterbacks often talk about the game "slowing down" as they become more experienced. For example, Drew Brees, quarterback of the New Orleans Saints, is famous for his high completion per-centage in which he will go through a number of "reads" before finding the open receiver.

Although some sports are not covered explicitly in this book, the reader can adapt the techniques presented here to work with any athlete. As will be shown in subsequent chapters, if the sport or event is one in which the therapist is not already proficient, of critical importance is communicating with the client's coach, when possible, regarding the specific concepts that he or she is attempt-ing to instill in the athlete.

Chapter 10 deals with recovering from injury and returning to competition, and Chapter 11 with substance abuse and other addictive behaviors among athletes. I recently published in the area of hypnosis with addictions (Tramontana, 2009a), so it fits in well for me to use these techniques with athletes. For any sports psychologist working with such issues, some grounding in addic-tions treatment would be helpful as well as some experience in the field of pain management. In the Conclusion, there are further suggestions regarding the generalization of these techniques and strategies for other areas in which peak performance is the goal.

In addition to hypnotic techniques, which might include age regres-sion and future projection, I use cognitive behavioral approaches, reframing and other neurolinguistic programming techniques, systematic desensitization, guided imagery and meditation, and *uncovering* psychodynamic reasons for lack of success. These meth-ods are employed both in and out of trance.

I have included numerous interviews in the book, such as with former National Football League player Brian Kinchen (Chapter 6), the former tight end and long snapper who snapped the ball for the New England Patriot's winning field goal in Super Bowl XXXVIII. Brian was the subject of *The long snapper* (Marx, 2009), which focused on the mental turmoil he faced preparing for that game after being out of football for three years. Other interviews are with Leaf Boswell, Louisiana State University (LSU) equestrian coach (Chapter 5), Yvette Girouard, LSU women's softball coach (Chapter 7); and Tony Minnis, LSU women's tennis coach (Chapter 8). Coach Minnis was recently selected to coach the Southern US team in the national tournament for high school girls sponsored by the United States Tennis Association in August, 2010. In 2009, he coached the Southern team to its first championship in 12 years. His comments about the mental side of tennis are especially relevant for anyone working with competitive tennis players. I interviewed him because I had not previously worked with any tennis players and wanted to get some inside information in order to develop some protocols. The same was true for my interview with the softball coach, Yvette Girouard. As a result of these two interviews, I have already gotten a referral from Coach Minnis and expect some from Coach Girouard in the future. Coach Boswell has already referred one of her riders as discussed in Chapter 5. The reader will note that time was spent in each interview educating the coach, to some extent, on how hypnosis works. The goal of this instruction is that in addition to getting information from the coaches about their particular sport, I wanted coaches to feel comfortable about making referrals to me and confident that hypnosis training can be of benefit.

Readers will receive the greatest benefit if they read the entire book rather than just individual chapters addressing their particular sport because there is much crossover of information and, in several places, you will be referred backward or forwards to another chapter. For example, in Chapter 6 (Football, Baseball, Basketball), there is an interview with football player Brian Kinchen on the 2003 Super Bowl, but little did I know beforehand what an avid and competitive golfer he is, nor how much of the interview he would spend talking about golf.

Chapter 2 includes a description of a telephone consult I had with a young golfer between his first and second days of competing in a world championship tournament. More recently, I had two telephone consults with the equestrian referred by Coach Boswell. These experiences proved very fruitful and have encouraged me to work with other athletes traveling to compete in other states or countries.

The reader will note a series of dots in the scripts (e.g., "..."). These dots represent what I believe to be strategic pauses in the delivery of the script for emphasis and/or to allow the client time to process what is being said to them. Of course, therapists can modify or adapt pause points to fit more easily with their own personal styles.

A special note: If an athlete's name is mentioned in the case examples, I have received written consent to do so. These are athletes I have worked with in the past; they are no longer clients, and no longer competing. This fact is important, as I do not wish to create a dual relationship in which an endorsement is given by a current client who then would serve as a marketing agent as well as a client.

Chapter 1

Overview of Hypnotic Approaches with Athletes

Whether you think yourself a success, or you think
yourself a failure, in either case, you're correct!

Anonymous

This quote is one of my favorites for all clients, not just athletes. Although the source is unknown, it sounds a lot like the work of Napoleon Hill in his book *Think and grow rich* (1938). Much of Hill's work is about meditation and focusing on what you would like to see happen in the future (in business, finance, life). Hypnotherapists refer to this as "future projection" or "rehearsing future success."

I anticipate that readers of this book will be different than those who have read my *Hypnotically Enhanced Treatment for Addictions* (2009), so some of the material on induction and trance deepening is repeated here. The strategies and techniques I use for entering hypnosis are the same regardless of the application.

One of the first issues I deal with when I first see an athlete – whether an adult who is a self-referral, but especially for young athletes who have been encouraged to see me by their parents – is to differentiate between psychotherapy and sports psychology. I explain:

> While I am trained as a clinical psychologist, in no way does the fact that you are seeing me imply that anyone thinks you have a mental or emotional problem. Clinical psychologists often see people with mental or emotional problems, addictions, or other behavioral problems *(the kids typically know someone with attention deficit hyperactivity disorder who had to see a psychologist)*. But sports psychology is a sub-specialty of psychology that does not

involve these problems. So I'm not going to be your "shrink" as some people call it. Rather, I would like you to think of me as your mental coach.

One exception was a professional golfer (see Chapter 2) who was referred by a colleague who diagnosed him with generalized anxiety disorder and obsessive-compulsive disorder. My colleague felt that hypnotherapy could help him with his clinical issues, but the client also wanted me to work with him on hypnotically enhanced achievement of peak performance. We decided we would focus on the clinical issues first, then later on golf.

While I spend time explaining hypnosis to all my clients, I believe a good orientation to hypnosis and self-hypnosis is especially important with the athlete-client. My reasoning is that the athletes spend so much time being coached on the mechanics of their respective sports that I want them to get a feel for the mechanics of hypnosis. I start by explaining that I think of hypnotherapy as involving two components: First, hypnosis is the art of getting the client (or self for self-hypnosis) into a hypnotic state and second, the therapy component involves what is done once the individual is in hypnosis. This represents the lens through which I see hypnosis working, as I understand it, and how I explain it to my clients.

When clients first come into my office, we discuss their presenting problems and determine the goal they wish to achieve. In this phase of information gathering, I especially like two questions recommended by Smith (2009) for beginning to work with athletes:

1. What percentage of your success is mental?
2. What percentage of your time do you spend on the mental part of your competition?

I tell athletes the same story I relate to all my new clients, although it is perhaps even more significant for them because I use a coaching metaphor that came out of a session with a new client.

> A number of years ago, I had a young man come in for his first psychotherapy session. I noticed from his information sheet that he had not been in therapy before. He was kind of fidgety and shuffling his feet. I asked him if he felt a little uncomfortable being

there. He said: "Yeah man, I don't know if I'm wasting your time and mine." I responded: "I know, guys are supposed to solve their own problems, right?" He agreed, and I continued, "And big boys don't cry, right?" Again he nodded in agreement.

Well, luckily for me, it happened to be that time of year, which happens every four years, when the Summer Olympics were going on. Coincidentally, the Summer Olympics are on the same four-year rotation as the presidential campaigns for the November elections, so the races were heating up. I asked: "Did you read the newspaper today?" After he acknowledged that he had, I asked: "Did you read about the Olympic athletes?" He responded: "Oh, yes. I love the Summer Olympics. I can't wait to get home from work every evening to watch them on TV." I continued: "Did you read about all of the presidential candidates? I'll bet everyone you read about who was good at anything had someone working with them behind the scenes to get better. The athletes all have coaches. The candidates have advisers, campaign managers, and speech writers. Actors and actresses have directors. Anybody who is good at anything has someone helping them get better."

Mike Tyson was heavyweight champion before he got so crazy and started biting people's ears off. But even Mike had this little old guy in his corner reminding him to keep up his left, move, and so on. Mike already knew he had to keep up his left, but sometimes it helps to have someone objective looking in and giving guidance. And that is how I see therapy. It is like having a coach, but one who coaches or consults with you regarding life's issues or problems you want to change.

This metaphor worked so well with that client that I began using it with others. The idea of a mental coach is accepted particularly well with adolescents, as well as adults, and it is not gender-specific. With athletes, I often modify the ending of the story – since we are not speaking metaphorically, but rather directly, regarding them seeing me as their coach in the mental aspects of their game.

Another topic I stress in the first session is the importance of being open. This discussion is perhaps less necessary with the athlete than with clients with addictions or other psychological issues, but I explain it to them anyway.

The therapist has only as much power to help as you give to him or her. And the way you give this power is by being honest and open. You know the old saying, "I can't fix it if I don't know what is broke"? Now I know it is sometimes hard to open up to a total stranger, but for me to help I have to know what I am really dealing with. A number of years ago, when I was director of a mental health center, I had an employee who was going through a divorce and needed therapy. She was also a friend. So I referred her to one of the psychiatrists who worked in one of our satellite clinics. I never breached privacy by asking her how the treatment was going, but one day curiosity got to me and I asked: "Are you still seeing Dr X?" She responded: "It is interesting you should ask, as we just had our final session last week." I asked: "Well, did it help?" She answered: "Oh, I don't know – not really." I expressed surprise: "Really, I always heard he was such a good therapist!" Her reply told the whole story: "Well, you know, Joe, that man never did know me!" I responded: "You mean you went to see that man once a week for six months and didn't let him get to know you?"

When a client wonders whether he or she can be hypnotized, my standard answer is: "Oh, anybody bright and creative can be hypnotized." Not surprisingly, the client typically accepts this perspective. I tell the client: "Only once has a client called my bluff, stating, 'Oh well, I guess that leaves me out!' As it turned out, she was a very bright (and witty) woman, and she was an excellent hypnotic subject." This response typically brings a chuckle from the client, thus enhancing rapport.

Regardless of why the client wants to be hypnotized – whether for performance enhancement, to quit smoking, lose weight, deal with other addictions, pain control, as an adjunctive technique to other psychotherapy, or something else – I always start off by providing an overview. Even if the client has been hypnotized by someone else in the past, this summary presents my particular philosophy about hypnosis and how it works. Typically, when describing to the patient what hypnosis is, I often find myself talking about what it is not. I tell the client:

Many people only have the image of stage hypnotists who try to convince spectators that they can use hypnosis to control the minds of individual members of the audience, even have them do silly things like crawl around like a chicken and cluck! But in medical and psychological hypnosis, the idea is that I cannot control your mind, nor would I want to. But I can teach you to use your own mind power to achieve your goals. The key is that it is your mind power, not mine, and your goals, not mine. So I serve only as a teacher or guide. You can't be hypnotized against your will, so we say that all hypnosis is self-hypnosis in a way. You have to be a willing participant. You have to want to do it.

Hypnosis is an altered state of consciousness. It is not an unconscious state. The name is a misnomer. It comes from the Greek word *hypnos*, which means sleep. But you will not be asleep, you will be very much awake. Your eyes will be closed only to block out distractions, just like the music lover might put on headphones and close his or her eyes to focus more intently on the audio and block out visual distractions. You will hear everything I say. You will be able to talk back if I ask you questions. You will remember everything we talk about, unless there is some reason to block it out. When your mind and body are totally relaxed, you can concentrate better on everything I say, on whatever we are dealing with, in this case suggestions about sports performance.

I typically add to this description of hypnosis by giving the client one or two brochures. The first, which I have used for years, is *Questions and answers about clinical hypnosis*. It was prepared by William Wester, a long time faculty member of the American Society of Clinical Hypnosis (ASCH), and can be purchased from Ohio Psychology Publications. The other, which I only started using recently, is *Hypnosis: what it is and how it can make you feel better*, and is published by Division 30, Society of Psychological Hypnosis, of the American Psychological Association. I then use the following techniques to orient the client to hypnosis.

Hypnotic suggestibility test

With athletes, one difference from my general hypnosis clients is that I always perform a test of hypnotic suggestibility and a muscle testing demonstration. The test of hypnotic suggestibility is as follows: I tell the client: "This is not hypnosis, but rather a test of visual imagery, since so much of our work will deal with visualization." Before starting, I demonstrate how they should hold out their arms at about shoulder height when I ask them to. Then, I say:

> Close your eyes. Settle back and relax. Now, I want you to imagine sitting on a beach, on a beautiful spring or summer day. Perhaps sitting on a beach towel or blanket or a recliner, and enjoying the beautiful weather. You feel the warm sunshine on your skin. There is a nice breeze coming off the water. You are just really enjoying the weather and the scenery. And I want you to imagine there are some children playing nearby, near the water's edge. Little children, perhaps children you know or they could be total strangers, and they are playing with their little sand buckets and shovels.
>
> Now when I was a kid, these buckets were usually made of some metal material, tin or aluminum. Nowadays they are typically plastic or rubberized. But they all have one thing in common, the little curved handle so the child can carry the bucket. And I want you to imagine that one of these children comes over to you and asks you to put out your arms. So go ahead and do so, as I showed you before. And imagine the child then places the bucket over the top of one of your wrists, so that it is hanging from that wrist. Then the child starts filling the bucket with sand. And as the child does so, the bucket becomes heavier and heavier. The natural pull of gravity will cause that bucket to feel heavier. And as it gets heavier, that bucket will gradually cause that arm to descend down towards the ground – the sand below. It is getting really heavy, and you would like to hold it up for the child, but you feel it getting heavier and heavier. It is about one-third full and getting really heavy. And now the child starts filling it with wet sand, and wet sand is even heavier than dry sand because it is denser. It is getting about half full, and now really heavy.

By this time, the arm has typically descended somewhat, and I tell the client: "Now, open your eyes and look at your arms." Occasionally, their arm has not descended, but they will report something like "It is really sore from holding up that bucket."

Muscle testing demonstration

> When I tell you to put out your arm, I want you to hold out one arm (the one closer to me), and after I describe something to you, I want you to make it very rigid and resist to the best of your ability when I try to push your arm down. Now, I want you to think about the greatest accomplishment in your whole life – something you are totally proud of that you would be happy for everyone to know about. You would be happy to see it published on the front page of the local newspaper. Nod when you have something in mind.

This typically does not take very long, and when they nod, I say: "Now resist." Invariably, the client shows great power to resist their arm being pushed down. Then they are told to relax the arm for a while, after which he or she is told:

> Now, I want you to think about the lowest, most lowdown thing you have ever done in your life, something you did that you should not have done or something that you should have done but didn't – something you are totally embarrassed about that you would not want anyone to know about. Nod when you have that in mind. Now make your arm rigid again, keep that negative thought in mind, and resist when I try to push your arm down.

Invariably, the client's arm is easily pushed down with this imagery. I then tell them a story about when I used this technique as a demonstration to the athletic department at the University of New Orleans. The story goes:

> I had worked with a varsity volleyball player who after just three sessions had her best game ever. *(This case is presented in Chapter 9).* She was written up in the local newspaper as having her career high in "digs." I didn't even know what a dig was but soon found out that it was a defensive save. When the coaches learned that I had taught her self-hypnosis, they invited me to give a presentation to the athletic department. I used this technique, asking for a volunteer from the audience. The women's basketball coach volunteered. He was not only tall but very muscular. I whispered the first instruction (regarding thinking something you are very proud of) in his ear. I then practically hung from his arm and could not budge

it. Then I whispered the negative suggestion, and this time his arm went down immediately and easily.

The goal is to instill confidence in the hypnotic approach by showing the client that he or she is likely to be a good hypnotic subject. I tell athletes an additional story:

> For five years I coached marathon teams for the Leukemia and Lymphoma Society's fund-raising campaign called Team-in-Training. The runners would raise money for treatment and research; and in exchange for raising X amount of money, the society would pay their travel, hotel, and entry fees to a marathon, usually in some really nice place to visit like Disney World, San Diego, San Francisco, Bermuda, or Maui, and would provide a running coach.
>
> Well, I was the coach for the Mississippi Gulf Coast Team for five years, and took runners to approximately 15 different marathons. These entrants had varying degrees of running experience, from veteran marathoners to first-timers. We would have a team run every Saturday, but in-between, they were to train on their own or in smaller groups, following a training schedule I had prepared for them. *Runner's World Magazine* was one of the sponsors and donated training logs. The runners were instructed to keep a weekly record of their running, for example, number of miles, conditions, and any cross-training. And at the bottom of each page was a quote. Now you know that there are many quotes about running that have to do with life in general. Probably the best-known one is: "Life is a marathon, not a sprint." You have heard that one before, haven't you? Well, one week, the quote was as follows: "Whether you think yourself a success, or you think yourself a failure, in either case, you're correct!" When I read that, I thought how much that applied to my general psychological practice, but perhaps even more specifically to athletes.

First hypnotic session

Induction and deepening

The first hypnotic session is often not until the actual second meeting. I feel it is very important to orient the client to what we are doing and why, so the first hypnotic session is highly structured and includes a series of specific techniques. I often start with a reverse arm levitation induction, followed by deep breathing techniques, and a deepening method involving the visual imagery of an elevator ride to a safe comfortable room.

I tend to use different induction and deepening techniques in subsequent sessions, including eye fixation, an eye roll approach, and progressive relaxation (imagined, not via progressive relaxation exercises). After the first three sessions, as clients become more experienced in my approach, I will often use what I refer to as "flex induction" during which I allow the client to choose which of the previously used induction and deepening techniques seemed most useful for them. In such cases, the client is told:

> You have been practicing a variety of induction techniques here and at home. Some clients prefer some methods and others prefer others! Now, just put yourself into a hypnotic state using whatever technique you like best. I have come to realize that for some clients just sitting in my recliner has become a conditioned stimulus to induce hypnosis.

In the first issue of the *American Journal of Clinical Hypnosis*, the founding editor, Milton Erickson, described what he referred to as "naturalistic techniques of hypnosis" (Erickson, 1958). He noted the importance of adequately meeting the client as a personality and his or her needs as an individual. My methods begin in a formalized way but evolve into a consideration of the client's needs and preferences. This continues to develop by asking the client: "What would you like (or what do you feel we need) to work on today in hypnosis?"

Sometime after completing the writing of my first hypnosis book, I came across an article that I had published years earlier (Tramontana, 1983). This case study, which focused on the importance of subject bias in hypnosis with children, reinforces the philosophy of letting the client choose the induction once they have been introduced to a number of options. The subject in this case was a 6-year-old thumb sucker. I noted that although I routinely question adults and adolescent clients regarding their knowledge of hypnosis, only a laconic and perhaps perfunctory discussion was entered into with this child because of his young age. Over a period of several weeks, I attempted to induce hypnosis with several of my usual techniques. Although the subject cooperated slightly and to varying degrees, his distractibility resulted in instances of interrupting to ask questions, opening his eyes to check on the therapist, and so on. Finally, after several failures to get him into a hypnotic state, he informed me: "You aren't doing it right." He had seen someone hypnotized on his favorite TV program, *Knight Rider*. He explained that in the show the hypnotist used a swinging watch. I improvised by tying the string from a tape recorder to my stopwatch to produce a pendulum effect. Once I did it "the right way" (according to the subject), a moderately deep hypnotic state resulted.

While athlete clientele seen for sports hypnosis are certainly much more sophisticated and informed than that young child, I sometimes tell this story to clients to let them know why I think it is important to allow them to choose techniques, especially for their self-hypnotic work.

Various deepening techniques are also employed. If I use the imagery of an elevator ride the first time, I might use a staircase, escalator, or gently sloping hill in subsequent sessions, always counting down. Later, I might use counting forwards as they imagine an elevator ride up into the clouds, each number taking them to a higher level of relaxation – *Where you can be above the humdrum of daily living and see things from a better perspective*. Again, after the client has become experienced in my deepening techniques, I will do the same as with the induction:

> You have also been practicing a number of different deepening techniques both here and at home, so you can pick whichever one you like best and allow yourself to go deeper now. Nod your head when you have completed the deepening technique in your mind.

The sessions typically go from structured, detailed approaches to shorter, less detailed and more flexible ones. I prefer the reverse arm levitation induction in the first hypnotic session because this approach is slower and more dramatic than some of the alternatives. While I am telling the client what is likely being felt in the arm and in the eyes, he or she is actually feeling the natural physiologic response of the arm and the eyes getting heavier. The ensuing more flexible and less detailed approaches are especially important for athletes since very early on they will be instructed in quick, open-eyed (alert) hypnosis for their competition.

The elevator

After hypnosis is elicited with the reverse arm levitation technique, some time is spent with diaphragmatic breathing. Then the client is told:

> Now, to get you more deeply relaxed, we are going to use a technique called visual imagery. Visual imagery is what we did in our first session when you imagined the beach scene. Some people refer to this as visualization. I sometimes call it getting a picture in your mind's eye. Almost as if you had a screen back behind the eyes and the mind could see it.

Since the client had previously experienced the beach scene imagery in my test of hypnotic suggestibility, I might reference that again:

> Just like with the beach scene, you demonstrated that you are good at visual imagery.

Following such confirmation, the client is presented with the next step:

> I want you to imagine yourself on the tenth floor of a building. This could be a building you have been in before or it could be one you have seen in a movie or on TV. But imagine that there are ten floors. You are on the top floor, and you want to take an elevator ride all the way down to the bottom floor. Each floor, as you go down, is going to symbolize or represent to you a deeper level of hypnotic

relaxation. I want you to use your senses. See yourself, feel yourself, sense yourself going deeper with each number as I count. Starting with the tenth floor, imagine you are standing in front of the elevator doors, the doors open and you step inside ... You turn around and face the front, and you will see a control panel with ten buttons, one for each floor, plus a couple of others for opening and closing the doors. Let me know by nodding your head gently when you get a picture in your mind's eye of that control panel ... *(If the client has difficulty, they are told to think about the last elevator they were in).* Now, I want you to imagine pushing the button that says one, and nod when you have done so ... Good, you have pushed the button that said one and you are ready to start your descent. You may notice above the doors often there is a set of lights and numbers, some way of monitoring your trip. But you have pushed the button and are ready to start down. Going down, from the tenth floor down to nine ... Deeper to eight *(I pace the counting with each exhalation of the client's breathing. This pacing should result in the client slowing down the breathing as I then start counting more slowly)* ... At seven going deeper. Every muscle and fiber in your body relaxing further and deeper with each number as I count ... Six and deeper ... At five you are halfway down and with the remaining numbers letting go of all remaining tensions and relaxing very deeply ... At four ... Three and deeper ... Two... All the way down to one, relaxing deeply.

And as you get to the bottom floor, imagine the elevator doors opening and you step into a hallway or corridor, and from there into a room ... A very warm, safe, peaceful, comfortable room. This could be a room you have been in before. It might even be your favorite room. Or it could be one you've seen in a movie or maybe in a magazine. Let me tell you how I see the room, and then you can either adopt my model or create your own. I see it as warm, safe, peaceful, tranquil. Perhaps thick carpet on the floor, and a couch or easy chair, the kind you just sink down into and feel almost like you are a part of the furniture ... See yourself entering the room, however you see it in your mind's eye, and walking over to the couch, or chair, or bed, or pillows, whatever furnishings are there, and really settling in, sinking in, becoming so deeply relaxed that it's hard to tell where your body stops and the furnishings beneath you begin. And if you allow yourself, you can become just that relaxed right here, in this chair *(or couch)*.

So deeply relaxed it's hard to tell where your body stops and the chair beneath you begins … As you appreciate how relaxed you're becoming … Appreciate how relaxed you've become … In a state of perfect relaxation, you feel unwilling to move a single muscle in your body. And feel how good it feels to know that you don't have to move a single muscle in your body.

The practice effect and generalization effect

Next, the client is instructed:

I'm going to tell you some things about hypnosis. You don't have to concentrate on what I am saying, because your subconscious will pick it up anyway. I'm going to tell you about two effects. First, the "practice effect." Just like most other behaviors, just as in your performances, the more you practice, the better you get. So let me suggest to you that anytime you want me to put you into a hypnotic state, you will go into hypnosis more quickly and more deeply (*I typically repeat the suggestion three times and state to the client that three is that magic number that "locks it in"*).

And the same thing will hold true with the self-hypnosis that I will be teaching you to practice at home. With practice, you will get better at putting yourself into a hypnotic state more quickly and more deeply. The key word here is the word "want." I said: "When you want me to put you into hypnosis." Neither I nor anyone else can put you into a hypnotic state against your will, and neither will you ever spontaneously go into a hypnotic state, for example, while operating machinery or driving a car (*unless the client is below driving age*). You will do so only when you want to, only when it is to your advantage to do so.

The second effect is what I call the "generalization effect." (*This effect is really an ego-strengthening approach, which I find to be especially important to athletes. The approach I use is to some extent a synthesis of Gregg's (1973) "*Analeptic circle*" and Hartland's (1966) ego-strengthening techniques.*) What I mean by generalization effect is that regardless of why you are learning hypnosis, whether it is to improve sports performance, stop smoking, lose weight, lower subjective levels of pain, decrease stress, overcome addictions, improve study habits … you see, there are many applications of hypnosis … the one common denominator or common fringe benefit, as I call it, is that you learn to be calm and more relaxed. Because that is what the hypnotic state is all about, learning to be more calm and relaxed … And when you learn to be more calm and relaxed, your functioning becomes more efficient and more effective. And as you function more efficiently and effectively, your self-confidence improves, leading to more calm and more relaxation, even more efficiency and effectiveness, and even more self-confidence.

Efficiency and effectiveness

With athletes, the goal is to reinforce a positive or optimistic forecast of success. The importance of efficiency is explained further, as follows:

Many people, perhaps most people, expend much too much emotional energy, much more than the particular situation calls for. This is what I call "spinning your wheels," emotionally. And I'm sure you are familiar with this metaphor, like a car stuck in mud. You rev the engine, and the wheels spin, but you don't go anywhere because you have no traction. As you learn to be more calm and relaxed, you will engage in less of that emotional wheel-spinning, and thus your functioning will become more efficient and more effective. And as you learn to function more efficiently and effectively, your self-confidence improves, leading to even more calm and relaxation, efficiency, effectiveness, self-confidence, and so on in a cycle of progress that grows, deepens, strengthens, and reinforces itself. This cycle of progress is like the so-called snowball effect. The little ball of snow that rolls down a hill and gets larger and larger as it gathers more and more snow. The end result of this cycle of progress is that you will have a better self-image, a better self-concept, what we call higher feelings of self-esteem. *(I don't say increased ego strength anymore, because I realized that some people who are not informed about psychology think that ego is a "bad thing" as in being too self-centered or having an inflated ego.)*

In other words, you will like yourself better, and you will be convinced that you can accomplish not only those things that you feel that you need to accomplish from day to day, but just about anything, within reason, that you set your mind to accomplish. And you will be able to do so calmly and relaxed, effectively and efficiently, with confidence.

Trance ratification

After the generalization effect, I focus on trance ratification. As noted by Hammond (1990, p. 19), trance ratification is vitally important in creating a sense of expectancy in the client. This experience provides the client with a convincer that ratifies for them that they have entered into an altered state of consciousness. He describes glove anesthesia (p. 20) as one such technique. While I use glove anesthesia with pain patients to demonstrate to them their ability to lower subjective pain, I do not typically use this with other hypnosis applications. Sports hypnosis is an exception, especially if the athlete is experiencing pain from an injury that might impede performance. With most other clients, I use the following three ratification techniques:

> Earlier I told you that you did not have to concentrate, because your subconscious would pick it up anyway. But now, I am going to ask you to do just the opposite, because I want you concentrate very intently on what I am saying. I want you to use the power of your creative mind, your imagination. And the first thing I want you to use your creative mind to imagine is that your eyes are glued closed. Almost as if you had accidentally gotten some Super Glue or Krazy Glue or some such substance on the lids or lashes and you cannot open them ... Now as you imagine your eyelids glued shut, let the muscles in your eyes try to open them, but your mind is telling you that you cannot open them because they are glued shut ... Notice the resistance. *(It has been very rare that a client opened his or her eyes.)* Mind over matter, mind over body. Now stop trying to open them. Imagine that the glue has worn off but you decide to keep them closed until later, when I tell you to open them.
>
> Now, I want you to place one arm out in front of you just like we did with muscle testing. I am going to touch your arm. Nod if that is okay? *(I then help them line up the arm directly in front of them*

25

at shoulder height.) Make it very rigid … That's right, make a fist and make the arm very rigid, like a bar of steel, an unbendable bar of steel. You might even form a picture in your mind's eye of a bar of steel there instead of an arm, tight and taut and unbendable *(I stroke the arm with my fingers and touch fingers around the wrist to demonstrate).* And now, as your mind tells you that is an unbendable bar of steel instead of an arm, let the muscles of the arm try to bend it. And notice the resistance there … Very good. Now I want you to imagine that the arm is no longer a bar of steel. Instead, it is like a dishcloth *(I put my fingers around wrist lightly).* Limp and loose like a dishcloth.

The arm typically flops down beside the client. In fact, their response to this exercise is one of the factors I consider when determining the client's hypnotizability or depth of trance. If they just gently lower the arm, it may be that they are going along with what they think I expect. If the arm drops like a dishcloth, this response indicates to me that they are truly in (or entering) into a hypnotic state. Then, depending on the particular application, appropriate suggestions follow.

The beach scene

Since so much of the first session is spent with goal-setting and orientation to hypnosis, there is not much time left for suggestions regarding their sport. But I want the client to leave that first session with something positive and encouraging to remember, so I tell them:

Now let's concentrate on getting even more deeply relaxed. We are going to do this by having you imagine some relaxing scenes. The first scene I want you to imagine is a beach scene, or if not a beach, perhaps on the ocean so you could be on the sand or grass, but I want you to imagine yourself sitting on a beach towel, a blanket, or a recliner of some sort and really enjoying the weather, the scenery. Perhaps it is a beautiful spring or summer day. Feel the warm sunlight on your skin, with a nice breeze coming off the water. You are really enjoying the weather and the scenery, watching some sailboats off in the distance. It is a relatively calm day and you notice how effortlessly they seem to move through the water, pushed by the gentle breeze. Perhaps there are some seagulls fly-ing nearby, near the water's edge, and you notice how they, too, seem to glide so effortlessly on the wind currents, and perhaps a ship on the horizon ... Now we know that it takes a lot of power to propel a ship, but it is the efficient use of power that causes this seeming effortlessness ... Perhaps a jet plane in the sky. It too takes a tremendous amount of power, but once again, it is the effi-cient use of power that causes this seeming effortlessness. These are your key words, "efficiency" and "effortlessness."

The woods scene

Now let's go to a second scene. This could be a scene in the woods, perhaps a state park-type setting. It is a beautiful fall morn-ing, one of those fall mornings where there is a nice sunlight, but you feel that certain crispness in the air. And you are walking down a path in the woods, really enjoying the scenery. The leaves are turning colors, birds are chirping, and you are enjoying the sights and sounds and smells of the forest. And as you are walking along the path, you notice an area ahead in which there are no trees. As you get closer you see the reason that there are no trees is that there is a body of water running through there, like a narrow river or wide stream, and you notice how effortlessly the water seems to flow, clean and clear ... It is so crystal-clear you can see your image, your reflection, in the water. And you might see your reflec-tion as you were at some younger age, some earlier time, when everything seemed easier, when you were more happy-go-lucky ... You notice how steadily the water flows, how predictably, reliably, efficiently and effortlessly ... There are those words again, efficiently and effortlessly. Perhaps there are some rocks and pebbles near the water's edge, where the stream is only an inch or two deep, and you notice how the water just kind of goes over or around these rocks or pebbles. Perhaps there are some boulders protruding out in the stream and you notice how there, too, the water just goes over or around and continues on its path, effortlessly.

You continue to walk along the bank of the river or stream and you come upon a bridge, a walking bridge, the kind you might see in a state park. A wooden bridge, with curved hand rails, some people call them footbridges. And you decide that you want to cross over to the other side. So you step up onto the bridge and start to walk across ... But as you get halfway across, you notice that something below has gone awry. The water below is getting muddy and dirty and backing up. It is not flowing so smoothly anymore. And as you look more closely, you see that what has happened is some logs were floating down this body of water and they got lodged under the bridge, causing a logjam. As you investigate even more closely, you see that there is one log that is bigger than the rest. It is the main problem. It has got wedged under the bridge causing the others to back up behind it. I want you to really concentrate on that big log ... Some people, when they concentrate on that big log, might imagine something written on that log ... written or engraved, or inscribed on that log. It might be a word or it might even be a name. It could be a sentence or even a full paragraph. It is not essential that you see something, but regardless of whether you do or not, what is most important is the next step.

You make a commitment to take matters into your own hands to free up the problem, to remedy the problem, and so you cross over to the other side and you find a board or a pipe or a tree limb, something you could use as a lever. And you set about the task of freeing up the logjam. Whether it involves leaning over from the bridge, leaning out from the bank, or even wading into the water, you use that board, pipe or tree limb as a lever to pry loose that big log. And to your surprise, with a little effort, it begins to loosen up, and as it loosens, it starts to float again under the bridge. And the other logs follow suit.

You go back up onto the bridge and you watch as the logs float off into the distance. And the farther away they get the smaller they seem, and the smaller they seem the farther away they are until they are so very far away they are like little tiny specks in the distance. And finally, they round a bend; you know they still exist somewhere, but they are no longer in your field of experience. You look back down into the water and you take great pride in the fact that the water is once again flowing smoothly, cleanly, reliably, predictably. You see your reflection again, but this time you see yourself at your present age, in the here-and-now, but you see yourself as looking much happier, like the younger person that you saw in the beginning, free from the worry ... And you take some pride in the fact that you took matters into your own hands to rectify, to remedy this problem.

Now, as you may have already figured out, this is a metaphor filled with symbolism. The body of water symbolizes your path through life and that is why we showed you at an early age, clean and clear and free … The little rocks and pebbles symbolize minor setbacks, minor frustrations. Of course the boulders represent bigger problems; the logjam, however, represents a major blockage, probably the issue that led you to seek treatment. Some people see something written on the log that might give them a clue … By the way, did you see something written on the log? *(If yes, find out what the person saw. If not, I continue)* … And some don't, as I said. Some might see a name, perhaps even their own name, suggesting that they are their own biggest problem, but the key is the decision to take matters into your own hands to free up the logjam … Which could be symbolic of your coming to see me. And perhaps I am, or hypnosis is, the lever, the board, the pipe, or tree limb. But in any event, once the main log is loosened, life begins to flow more smoothly again. And as you look down again from the bridge into the water, you see it again as clear and clean and flowing. You see your reflection again, but this time in the present time. And you may even be smiling. You might be proud that you took matters into your own hands to remedy the problem.

I believe the logjam imagery can be very effective with athletes to help in releasing blocks (some golfers refer to it as "yips"). The logs and the big log seem more directly related to what may be obstructing their success. As a result, the symbolism is even less subtle than with other conditions for which I use hypnosis.

Second hypnotic session

Eye fixation induction

In the second hypnotic session, the client is told:

Last time, we created tension in your eyes and in your arm. This time, we are going to localize the tension just in the eyes. So I want you to stare at X. *(In one office, I had a picture of a burning candle high up on the wall, and I had the client stare at the flame of the candle. In other settings, I might just tell the client to pick a spot on the wall or ceiling that necessitates that they look up at an angle.)* This time we are localizing the tension just in the eyes, and very quickly you will feel the eyes getting heavier and heavier ... This technique is called eye fixation, which is just a fancy way of saying staring. And this causes the eyes to get heavier and heavier. And whenever you are ready to let go of the tension in your eyes, all you need to do is close the eyes comfortably and gently and relax further all over.

Once again, the induction is followed by diaphragmatic breathing exercises, and then a different deepening technique. A typical breathing exercise is introduced:

I want you to take a really deep breath. Hold it ... And as you exhale, just feel the tensions escaping from your body ... Again, take a really deep breath. And now relax ... Breathing is a key to relaxation. One of the things we know about human behavior is that humans are most relaxed when they are in a really deep sleep, and during that deep sleep stage our breathing changes. It becomes very slow and very heavy. So I want you to breathe as you would in a really deep sleep, slow and heavy, slow and deep, and each time as you breathe in you might think, in with relaxation, out with tension ... Relax in ... Tension out.

If the elevator image was used in the first session, the imagery of descending a staircase would likely be used in the second session. The exception is if a client indicates a fear of elevators, which is rare (I have never seen it with athletes), then I typically use the staircase the first time and move up the sequence of other imagery in subsequent sessions.

The staircase

The client is told:

Last time, we used the image of an elevator ride; this time we are going to use a staircase. Perhaps it is a spiral staircase, or perhaps one of those majestic staircases like in old mansions, so long as each step symbolizes or represents to you a deeper level of hypnotic relaxation. I want you to use your senses. See yourself, feel yourself, sense yourself going deeper with each number as I count. Starting with the tenth step and going down. *(The patient is then taken from the tenth step all the way down to the first step.)*

Third hypnotic session

Eye roll induction

The third induction technique, which I usually introduce after the reverse arm levitation and eye fixation techniques have been utilized, is the eye roll. Again the goal is to teach the client a variety of methods so they can choose the one that seems to work most effectively for them. I often recommend the eye roll technique for self-hypnosis, as it can be done just about anywhere, even in public, by covering the brow with a hand. I tell them: "Others around you might think that you are just thinking or, at worst, have a headache. They do not have to know that you are putting yourself into hypnosis." The client is told:

> I want you to look up as if you are trying to look up through your eyebrows or your skull. And you will feel the tension very quickly when staring at this angle. Whenever you feel that tension really building and want to let go of it, just close your eyes gently and relax further all over.

The patient is told for both the eye fixation and eye roll techniques:

> We find that we can get more relaxed by creating tension in the eyes and then letting it go, than if we just say, "I think I'll close my eyes and relax now." It has to do with the difference between tension and relaxation, just like in the old progressive relaxation exercises in which people were taught to tense various muscles and then relax them. It is the contrast between tension and relaxation, which are mutually exclusive behaviors, incompatible responses, that teaches you to get more deeply relaxed. As therapists who teach progressive relaxation techniques typically say after a

particular muscle group is tensed and then relaxed, "notice the difference between tension and relaxation."

Subsequent sessions might entail deepening techniques such as an escalator ride or descending a gently sloping hill down to a beautiful valley or an ocean. When working with a client over several sessions, I often have them count forwards from 1 to 10 in an imaginary trip up into the clouds. Some clients have reported preferring this approach to counting down. They are told that from this vantage point, perhaps they will have a better perspective of things going on down below at ground level. I sometimes use this approach for creating a time continuum. The client can look to the left into the past (age regression), or to the right into the future (future projection). This flexible approach helps increase the client's repertoire of techniques that they can use in doing their own self-hypnotic work.

Alert and open eye hypnosis

With athletes, the alert or open eye trance is of particular benefit. They are told, for example:

> When you practice at home, just as here, you will have your eyes closed, but I will teach you techniques for getting into a trance state with your eyes open and fully alert. After all, you cannot compete any other way! There are many good examples of open-eyed trances in our daily living. For example, have you ever been so focused on a TV show or a book, or a computer game that someone could come into the room and speak to you but you really don't comprehend what they are saying? You were so focused on the show or book or game that you kind of blocked them out. Or perhaps *(if they are old enough to drive)* you were driving somewhere, to work, school, a social function, or maybe to your practice or competition, and you got there safely but do not remember the trip, whether you stopped for traffic lights, or little else? You were probably driving safely, but you were so focused on whatever you were thinking that you blotted out much of the drive. These are examples of open-eyed hypnosis or what I sometimes call mini-trances.

Edgette and Rowan (2003, pp. 73–83) discuss the importance of alert hypnosis, along with techniques of teaching this approach. I especially like Wark's (2009) method of implanting the expectation of increased ability to focus. For example, he poses the question: "Wouldn't it be nice to focus so well on ___?" (whatever the client's competition or event might call for). My technique is somewhat different because I start with closed eyes and then incorporate open-eyed hypnosis.

> We have been practicing hypnosis here, in my office, with your eyes closed in order to block out distractions. But, of course, you must have your eyes wide open and be totally alert when practicing or competing. So this is what you are to do: Before a practice or competition, put yourself into hypnosis, using the quickest and most effective way that works for you, and give yourself the following post-hypnotic suggestion. I am now (if you are doing this immediately before the event), or in X hours or minutes (if you are doing it the night before or morning of); and we will talk about a plan for you to use the hypnotic technique at all of these times, going to open my eyes and be wide awake, alert, rested, and energetic, and totally focused. Just as focused as when my eyes were closed, focusing totally and only on the task at hand.

Self-hypnosis

The client is told to practice at home. Starting at the end of the first hypnotic session, I teach a three-step self-hypnosis approach. The client is then given the instructions for eye fixation as described above (second session).

> Step one: Today I had you stare at a spot on your hand, localizing the tension in both your eyes and your arm. By next time, I will have you staring at a spot on the wall, localizing the tension just in the eyes. So this is what I want you to do at home. Stare at that spot, and when you decide to let go of the tension, just close the eyes and relax further all over. This is step one, creating the tension, and then letting it go.

> Step two involves the deep breathing as we described it today. Unless people have breathing problems, they tend to take breathing

for granted, but if you can spend two or three minutes getting into your own breathing, breathing slow and deep, it is like getting into yourself, blocking out distractions.

Step three involves counting down, from 10 to 1, as we did today. Whether it is an elevator ride, or descending a staircase or a gently sloping hill, each number takes you to deeper levels of relaxation. Then, you can review those things we worked on today. If you are doing this at bedtime, you might give yourself the post-hypnotic suggestion that you are going to fall into a deep and restful sleep, not to awaken until the appointed time. If you're doing this during the day and have other responsibilities, tell yourself: I will continue to relax for X minutes, whether it be 5 minutes, 30 minutes, or just 1 minute, depending on how much time you have to relax, after which time I will open my eyes feeling wide awake, relaxed, refreshed, calm, confident, and alert.

The particular application of hypnosis determines how many times per day a client is instructed to practice. During a Pulos and Smith (1998) workshop I learned that athletes are so used to practicing repetitions that they can be instructed to use self-hypnotic techniques many times a day. For example, Smith asked the workshop participants how many times a day they typically told their clients to practice. Most said two or three. He said he tells his athlete-clients to practice self-hypnosis 100 times a day. Many eyebrows went up. For example, if they are watching TV, he will advise them to use a quick hypnotic approach during every commercial, coming out of hypnosis as soon as the program comes back on. This also teaches them to move in and out of hypnosis very quickly, which is often very beneficial in their respective sports. Of course, I never tell clients to practice 100 times per day; typically, I tell them to do it several times a day.

Another difference between athletes and my standard clients is that I almost always make a recording for their home practice. With other hypnosis applications, I typically only record a session if the client reports having trouble getting into the hypnotic state when practicing at home. With athletes, unless they tell me that they do not need or want the recording, I do one. They are told that with practice they will depend less and less on the recording, because, of course, they will not have access to this equipment during their competition.

I also discuss with athlete-clients the theory that some stress might relate to alertness – for example, if an athlete is too relaxed they might not be able to perform at peak levels. Some writers on the subject say that peak performance is just below the point where anxiety begins (Saunders, 2005; Smith, 2009). I also tell my clients about something I learned from John Wolfe who, at the Yerkes Laboratories of Primate Biology during the 1930s, taught chimps to work for tokens which they could then use to secure food). He later became Chairman of the Psychology Department at the University of Mississippi. I remember well from graduate school that he taught us that you can never "unlearn" a behavior. Instead, you learn a new behavior that is incompatible with the old behavior. This idea seems especially relevant when working with athletes who have developed bad habits which are hurting their performance.

Inspirational stories

I find storytelling a very effective teaching technique with athletes (see Tramontana, 2009a,b,c). When clients hear a story about others, they often understand more clearly (and are less likely to be defensive) how the phenomenon might apply to them than if they are given direct suggestions. My favorite quote about storytelling comes from Dawn Daniels of Stone Soup Productions:

> I believe in the power of story to awaken, to challenge, to enrich, and to heal. Come sit by my fire.

I also tell athletes about famous sports stars who use self-hypnosis. For example, a professional football field-goal kicker who would go through a pre-kick ritual that involved a hypnotic approach and visualization of the ball going through the uprights. Interestingly, field-goal kicking is different than the rest of the game of football, because there is more time to think before kicking. That is why opponents will often call a timeout before a kicker attempts a clutch field goal. They call it "icing the kicker."

I also refer to inspirational movies about sport with athletes more than for any other client group. I'll often suggest that they watch the Kevin Costner movie *For Love of the Game*. I especially want them to see what he does to block out distraction, especially when playing in the opponent's ballpark. The home crowd is often very hostile. They heckle him and tell him what a bum he is, and so on. His ritual is to say to himself, "Clear the mechanism," and it is as if he suddenly becomes deaf, blocking out all sound. This approach is a form of self-hypnotic trance induction.

There are other movies about football and other sports that are very inspirational. For example, I remember a story about the coach of a college basketball team having his team watch *Remember the Titans*, which was a movie about a high school football team, but with an inspirational message that crosses all sports. For other inspirational movies about sports, see the Recommended Books and Movies at the end of the book.

Uncovering

If a client is having problems in their game that appear to be related to low self-esteem, self-sabotage, or some other emotional reason, I will do some uncovering work with them. This approach is initiated usually after the client has already had some experience with the hypnotic techniques described above. Prior to initiating an uncovering technique, and to give clients an example of the power of this approach, I tell them a story (out of trance), about a girl whose problem had nothing to do with sports; rather, it had to do with self-esteem:

> Years ago, when I was on rotation to do psychological testing at an adolescent psychiatric hospital, I was called to see a 16-year-old girl admitted to the unit. The nurse told me when I arrived: "This kid feels like she doesn't fit in, and she really doesn't. The other kids don't like her, and we don't like her." Well, they didn't actually admit that, but it was the impression I got. But, I liked her. She was a pretty girl but, of course, she thought she was ugly. A few days after completing the examination, I received a call from the unit nurse. She said: "Dr T, you are the only one who connected with this kid. Would you like to follow her on an outpatient basis when

she is discharged?" I replied: "Yes, but since I'm there a couple of days a week anyway, how about if I start seeing her as an inpatient, then at my outpatient office after discharge?" The hospital staff agreed.

In our first inpatient treatment session, I talked with her about this feeling of never fitting in. She admitted that she felt that way but did not know from where it originated. It was just always there. I talked with her about hypnosis (if her mom agreed), but noted it was too noisy there, with kids making noise in the hallways, the overhead speakers, and so forth, but I said we could do it when she came to my office.

In our very first outpatient session, hypnosis was begun. She entered a hypnotic state easily. I had her imagine watching a movie of her life, and told her as I counted backwards from 5 to 1 the film would rewind, and when we got to 1, a picture would come into focus on the screen that would tell us about some very significant experience in her past related to the problems she had in the present with not fitting in. When I got to 1, she told a story that had occurred when she was 3 years old. She said she had just gotten out of the bathtub, so she had no clothes on, and she was playing on the floor with her dolls. Her mother entered the room and severely berated her. She told her what a nasty, naughty little girl she was: "Shame on you, NAKED!" Tears were running down the child's face as she described this scene. I remember thinking, boy what a mean mother, but I'll bet that wasn't the first time something like that had occurred.

So I told her that I was going to count backwards again, and this time when I got to 1 I wanted her to tell me about the very first experience in her life that might relate to why she always felt that she didn't fit in. She described an incident when she was an infant. She didn't know how old she was, but knew that she didn't yet know how to talk but she could hear. She was in a baby crib, and she could hear her mother and her grandmother arguing in the next room. The grandmother was saying, "I told you that you should not have had that baby. Her father wouldn't marry you. There is no place for her in this world." At this point, she again cried profusely. That was the insight part of the technique.

Next, I wanted to re-program her thinking about these experiences. I said: "You know, it doesn't sound to me like you had a very nice grandmother. I know I surely don't like her. To say the least, she didn't seem to have the sensitivity or ability to love and accept you, and to cherish you the way you deserved. But what if you had the most wonderful grandmother in the world, one with all of the Christ-like (I don't do religious counseling, but I knew she was a Christian, so used it) qualities of love, and compassion, and empathy. What if you had that kind of grandmother? What would she have said?" Her tears turned to a big smile, and she offered: "She would have said, 'What a beautiful baby! I'm so glad we have her!'" To which I said: "And that is what most grandmothers would have said. Unfortunately, you were stuck with this mean-spirited grandmother who was incapable or unwilling to give you the love you deserve. But that's not your fault!

"Now let's go back to when you were 3 years old, playing naked on the floor with your dolls. If you had the most wonderful mother in the world, one with all of those Christ-like qualities, or better yet, if you were the mom and it was your 3-year-old daughter, what would you have said?" She responded: "I would have said: 'Honey, it's not good hygiene to play on the floor without any panties, so you can get dressed and play or you can get up in the bed and play.'" To which I asked: "You mean you wouldn't have told her she was a BAD GIRL?" She responded: "Of course not!" "Well, then, were you a bad girl?" I asked. And she responded: "OF COURSE NOT!" Once again, the idea was reinforced that it's not your fault!

The client is then told:

She left that day like a different person. Now, not in all cases in which we use uncovering work are the results so dramatic, or achieved so quickly, but this case gives you an idea about how things that happened long ago might have some impact on your life in the present.

To begin the technique, I tell the client:

As you continue to relax in this manner, I am going to teach you a technique to understand and let go of whatever it is that has been blocking you. If we can find an early origin of the problem that is blocking you from success, this creates what we call an "affect-bridge." By finding the origin, it bridges the gap, so to speak. And we are going to use a technique called hypnoprojection. I want you to imagine sitting in front of a giant screen, and in just a moment, as I count backwards from 5 to 1, imagine the film rewinding. And when we get to 1, a picture will come into focus on that screen. And that picture will tell you about some past experience in your life related to the problems in the present that are blocking you from being your best self. The reason we are using hypnoprojection is that by imagining watching a movie of your past, you do not have to re-live it, just in case there was something traumatic. Rather, you imagine that is a documentary and you are the narrator of that documentary. Only it is a documentary about your life.

Uncovering/regression is one the many strategies I utilize to assist the client in learning to understand the origins of self-sabotaging or self-handicapping behavior.

Reframing

Reframing is another technique that seems especially important for athletes. With golfers, for example, I might get them to think about errors, not failures, and how both errors and good shots are experiences from which we can learn. A story I often tell athletes is as follows:

A number of years ago I had an attorney who came to see me. He said that the night before a big trial, he would feel so much anxiety that he would prepare and over-prepare to the point that he did not get enough sleep and was thus not at his best when he got to court. Well, I knew from our history gathering session that he enjoyed sports and had, in fact, played football in high school. So I asked him if he remembered the feelings he had the night before and morning of a big game. He acknowledged that he did. I said that I'm sure then that he probably felt some butterflies in his stomach, but I'll bet that as soon as the action started they went away. He said that I was correct. So I asked: "So would you call those feelings, those butterflies, anxiety?" To which he responded "No, I don't know what I would call them, but definitely not anxiety." I said: "How about anticipation? Or excitement?" He said that yes, these were better descriptions of what he was feeling before a big game. I countered: "And that is what you are feeling the night before a big trial. Anxiety is a form of fear. You are not afraid. Just the opposite, you are ready to get on with the action, ready to rumble." Once this reframing had taken place and he saw his feelings as excitement, anticipation, or readiness, his response to the situation changed drastically. He reported later that the night before the next trial he had after that, he had "slept like a baby" and woke up alert and refreshed, and put on his "best game."

Cognitive-behavioral approaches

Much has been written about CBT, but one story I tell my clients about this approach is as follows:

I was teaching a night psychology class at the University of South Alabama. In those days, I had not yet learned hypnosis. I was discussing Albert Ellis and how he talked about how most people think that a particular stimulus situation, which we'll call A leads to B, which is the response or reaction. *(In the class I diagramed it on the blackboard; with clients I use a sheet of paper.)* But Ellis said this was not correct: The response is not B, but rather it is C. B is your belief system or what you tell yourself about A that causes C.

Well, it just happened that I had two police officers in the class who were working on a degree in Criminal Justice. They often came to class in uniform and always sat next to one another. One of the officers said: "Doc, I know what you are saying, but I disagree. I am a law enforcement officer and have a very stressful job. My doctor tells me that I now have a stomach ulcer because of stress. So it sounds like my job is A and my response is B, the ulcer." I asked him to describe his job. He said: "Well, we ride in a patrol car and people give us no respect. They call us words like 'pig.' People are shooting at us, and I am having trouble sleeping at night."

It appeared that his fellow officer was very calm and cool, so on a hunch I took a chance and called on him. I said: "Now the two of you are partners, right?" After his affirmation of this along with the fact that they ride in the same patrol car, I said: "So how about if you describe your job to the class." He responded: "Well, he's right. People often don't respect us. And they do call us names. One time, somebody threw a brick at the car." (Guy number one says they're shooting at them.) "But I don't lose any sleep over it. It's just a job." To which I responded: "Wait a minute! You don't lose any sleep over it and it's just a job – don't tell me you DON'T have an ulcer?" He answered: "Of course not." His partner with the ulcer said: "Screw you!" (to his partner, not to me, at least I don't think it was to me). So you see, what you tell yourself about the situation determines your reaction to that situation.

In this chapter, I have presented my general approaches to hypnosis, examples of induction and deepening techniques, as well as some of the general concepts I use when working with athletes. The following chapters zero in on treating athletes in specific sports, with some case examples which show how well these individuals usually respond to learning hypnotic techniques and applying them to achieve peak performance.

Each chapter begins with a motivational quote, some by famous people, others are anonymous. I use these as well as a number of similar quotes, as affirmations which I give to the client as a handout, so they can pick and choose which ones fit his or her situation best (see Appendix). This list includes selected quotes from a more comprehensive one that can be found at www.dennydavis.net/poemfiles/success.htm. The client is asked to pick the relevant ones and print them out in large bold letters to be pasted on their walls, mirrors, or lockers – anywhere that will remind them to "think success."

For those athletes who are actively competing, I often remind them of the song that Whitney Houston recorded for NBC's theme song for their production of the 1988 Summer Olympics in Seoul, South Korea entitled "One Moment in Time," written by Albert Hammond and John Bettis. The lyrics of this song very inspiringly reinforce the importance of seizing the moment, when it avails itself, to be the best that you can be, to excel, to do something great. I sometimes encourage them, if they seem to be the type to download tunes, to download it or perhaps just download the words which are very inspirational.

Yet another motivational event I sometimes refer to is the talk given to the New Orleans Saints football team by Ronnie Lott, the famous Hall of Fame defensive back, the night before their 45-7 shellacking of the Oakland Raiders in a preseason game in August, 2009. According to Saints quarterback Drew Brees: "Coach ran off all of his accolades, which are unbelievable and impressive." Brees added: "But, he told us that he'd trade it all to get one more chance to compete. Competitors always have that feeling. He talked about our window of opportunity and the sacrifice that we need to make as players for ourselves and the good of the team." Interestingly, this was the year the Saints went on to go to their first Super Bowl and win the world championship.

Chapter 2

Golfers

Life isn't about waiting for the storm to pass.
It's about learning to dance in the rain.

Vivian Greene

In the first draft of this chapter, I made the following statement: "Let me begin by noting that I have never worked with a champion or so-called elite golfer. I have, however, worked with golfers at many levels, including professionals, one of whom made the LPGA qualifying tournament, and another played for a couple of years on an Asian tour, and all of whom reported improved performance following the experience. This fact is likely to be especially pertinent to those golfers who are not professional, much less champions, but good enough to aspire to go professional or even to get better and to achieve peak performance while continuing to play at the amateur level." Since then, however, I have had the privilege of working with a young girl who won a world championship in her age group. This experience has been quite delightful because she is so motivated, dedicated, and insightful, and has the ability to generalize the techniques I have taught her from the golf course to the classroom.

Before getting into the specific techniques I use with golfers, I will present four case examples.

Case 1: The professional golfer

The first athlete I ever worked with was a professional golfer. He was referred to me in 1984 by a mutual acquaintance who was, in fact, one of his supporters and paid for his sessions with me. Despite the fact that this case was some 25 years ago and all of the files in my Mississippi Gulf Coast office were lost in Hurricane Katrina, I remember him well. His sponsor had given me a copy of Timothy Gallwey's *The inner game of golf* (1981), which I quickly read before the first session. The client told me that in every tournament qualifying round, he would do fine until the last hole or two, then he would "blow up" and miss the qualifying cut by one stroke. This reminded me very much of what Gallwey talks about regarding athletes creating their own obstacles to achievement.

The first session focused primarily on introducing him to hypnosis and relaxation training, as well as deep breathing methods, with suggestions on how to generalize these techniques for his golf game. In the second session, I felt it important to use hypnotic regression to uncover what was causing him to break down just before qualifying. He was regressed to his most recent tournament to review what thoughts were going through his mind just before the final hole. What came out was very interesting. He said that his sponsorship had basically run out. He had no funds, and he knew that if he qualified, he did not have enough money to even stay in a hotel and buy meals during the rest of the tournament.

What followed was not part of psychology or hypnotherapy! I called a good friend in New Orleans who was always very interested in golf and is a good amateur player, and who is now a committee member for the Zurich Classic in New Orleans. I explained the situation to him, and he arranged for my client to go to New Orleans and play with some of his businessmen golfing friends, who wound up sponsoring him for a while. We had another two hypnotic sessions during which I attempted to hypnotically reinforce some of the concepts I had learned from Gallwey's book. All the while, I explained that my focus was not on the mechanics of his game, which he already knew and whatever tweaking of which would be done by his golf coach, but the mental aspects. In his next tournament competition, which was a small, local one, he not only qualified but won first place money. He later gave me a few free golf lessons, and the next thing I heard was that he was on the Asian Tour.

As this experience was so long ago and I had no paper records, but I wanted to include my first case of using sports hypnosis in this chapter, I tracked him down recently. I explained that the reason I called was that I would like to include my work with him in a book and wanted to know if he felt the hypnotic experience had helped, and if so, how. One of the first things he said was: "My biggest mistake was not staying with you a little longer! The best I ever played was after we worked together a couple of times. The first few tournaments after that were the best I ever played! I had a 74.1 average in 1983 and 1984 and lowered it to 71.6 in 1985 and 1986.

He said that in the first tournament he won after seeing me, he remembered he would play a round and then "wake up" after the last hole: "I was focused on hitting the ball and then totally forgetting golf. You told me that whether the shot was good or bad, to focus on something else; the water if near an ocean, the trees, or birds. Anything but golf! I remember finishing several strokes ahead of the field on one round and not remembering the round because I was so focused."

I had learned this advice from Gallwey (1981). He describes how in tennis, a player is hitting a moving ball over and over again on the run or a skier is hurtling down a mountain, so their reactions are much more instinctual than mental. The golfer, however, has more time to think between shots. If the previous shot was a bad one, this thinking can involve grappling with self-doubt, anxiety, fear of failure, and tension. This difference is similar to the distinction between working with sprinters versus distance runners, as will be seen in Chapter 3. In most sports, too much time spent thinking about a good shot can also distract the player.

He added: "Back then, unless they were on the PGA Tour, few people could make enough money to survive, even on the Asian Tour." In 1987 he met a girl from Jackson, Mississippi, quit playing, got married, and started working as a golf pro, then began selling real estate, and is now a stock trader. He said: "It was tough quitting. I wish I had stuck with you longer." He then asked if I had watched the US Masters the previous weekend, adding: "Several of the leaders melted in the last two holes. They could have used your help!" The April 20, 2009 issue of *Sports Illustrated* featured an article by Alan Shipnuck entitled "Last man standing." The author discussed events and twists at the end of that Masters that led to Ángel Cabrera's victory. Interestingly, on the cover of that edition the strapline read: "The Masters: Angel and the Bedeviled."

In his (2009) article Hodenfield notes: "In the nerve-wracking game of pro golf, Nicklaus' method – which he talked about openly – was to do the very best he could against the course and just let the other guys fall apart like a cardboard suitcase. When the pressure was loaded on, they usually did." He reports that Tom Weiskopf, Nicklaus' long-suffering rival, said: "Jack knew he was going to beat you. You knew Jack was going to beat you. And Jack knew that you knew he was going to beat you." He adds: "Tiger is hearing the same music now."

Case 2: The college golfer

Lisette Lee (now Prieto) is a female golfer who was in the qualifying school for the LPGA. She saw me on two occasions in 2002. She had been an excellent college golfer and was selected for the All-SEC team in 2000. She was also SEC Athlete of the Week twice that year and had ten top 10 finishes. In 2000, she received the Dinah Shores Trophy sponsored by the LPGA Foundation. As a senior at Louisiana State University (LSU) she also received the Boyd McWhorter SEC Scholar-Athlete Award.

Once again, because I had lost my paper files in Hurricane Katrina, I interviewed her to ask about her recollections of our work together, if it helped, and, if so, how. When I talked with Lisette, she reminded me that she had also played in the US Open in 1996, the summer between her senior year in high school and her freshman year at LSU. She had married a caddie for a female golfer (who has since made it to the LPGA tour), who was now a teaching pro at a country club, and they had a 20-month-old son. She had not been competing or even playing very much but did remember vividly her two sessions with me almost seven years earlier.

She said at that time she had been on the LPGA futures tour from 2000–2003 with her best (a 12th place finish) in 2001. She added: "I was too focused on the money and put extra stress on myself."

JT: *Do you think the hypnosis training helped?*

LL: *Absolutely! I remember you counting me down, and an elevator, and a staircase. I remember using the techniques to bring my emotions, which there were a lot of, into a controlled state. Obviously it worked because I had tried to qualify for the LPGA tour in 2000 and in 2001 and never made it past the first stage. You helped me calm down and focus, and in*

2002 I made it to the finals. I remember the deep breathing exercises really helped me a lot, especially on the first hole. That first hole is probably the most nervous you'll ever be. For me, it wasn't the tee shot. It was the walk from the tee to the second shot of the first hole. That is when the deep breathing – you told me all the way from my stomach – calmed down my emotions.

JT: *Do you remember us talking about visualizing the next shot, then, when it was over, to let it go so thinking about the last shot, whether it was good or bad, would not interfere with the next one?*

LL: *Yes, I remember those two techniques. I had forgotten, but now that you mentioned them I remember using them. Visualization really helped. I would picture the shot before I hit it or even before my practice swing, and even visualize the flight of the ball.*

The mental part of golf is so important. That's why Tiger Woods is so much better than the others. Of course he is a good striker, but they all are. He is just so mentally good!

Case 3: The scholarship golfer

Yet another promising player was a young man who had just received a golf scholarship to a very prestigious Catholic, mid-western University. What I found to be especially significant about my experience with him was that he reported that after just a few sessions with me, he had achieved his lowest score ever. I had used many of the suggestions that Bob Rotella gives to his golfer clients, albeit while he was in a hypnotic state (he proved to be a good hypnotic subject). This struck me as significant because the client informed me that Bob Rotella was a family friend and he'd had some sessions with him – in which he was given many of the same suggestions conversationally – but that he had never played so well as after the hypnotic suggestions. This statement is in no way meant to be disparaging of Rotella, as he is a highly respected sports psychologist, and I have learned much from his books.

Case 4 : The professional golfer in emotional distress

This case is noteworthy because of the confluence of emotional distress along with this professional golfer's problems in competition. The first thing that needed treatment was his emotional difficulties. He certainly could not focus on his game when he was suffering from a clinically significant generalized anxiety disorder as well as a number of interpersonal and relationship problems. At the time of this writing, outcome information cannot be given since we are in the early stages of working on his emotional issues, and his next planned competition is a few months away.

My first task was to deal with his clinical anxiety. After discussing with him Selye's (1956) description of panic attacks (the so-called "fight or flight" response), I used a number of hypnotic approaches including a takeoff of the control room metaphor (which I also use with patients for lowering subjective pain). This method is a synthesis of Garver's (1990, p. 61) Control Switch Visualization for pain patients and Hammond's (1990, pp. 354–355) Master Control Room technique for patients with sexual dysfunction. The client is told:

> I want you to imagine that you can go into a place in your own brain … Perhaps if you've ever been to Disney World or is it Universal Studios, there was a ride in which you were in like a spaceship and you were projected inside the human body to see the heart, lungs, and so on. Let's suppose you could be projected inside your own brain. Your brain is the control center of your body, much like the NASA Space Center that we see in the movies. The astronauts are always communicating with Houston. So imagine you can go inside this control center, in your brain. The brain is, in fact, your control center … Imagine you come upon a lot of technical instruments. There are monitors, gauges, controls, and switches. And you see a monitor on the left which has a gauge for tension, stress, or anxiety … They all mean pretty much the same thing … And just to the right, there is a monitor for calm and relaxation … And let's imagine that at first, the level on the left gauge, tension or anxiety, is a 9 on a 10-point scale … And the one on the right, the relaxation scale, is a 1 … Imagine that you can then begin to adjust the levels … There are knobs, like rheostats … And as you turn up

the relaxation knob clockwise from a 1 to a 2 with your right hand, you turn the anxiety/tension knob down counter-clockwise to an 8 with your left hand … Next, you turn the relaxation gauge up to a 3 … And simultaneously turn the tension gauge down to a 7 … You continue turning the relaxation gauge up to a 4, but as you are about to turn the tension down to a 6, you notice a very interesting phenomenon … That knob seems to be turning by itself, automatically … And this is understandable, because tension and relaxation are incompatible responses. They are what we call mutually exclusive … You can't be tense when you're relaxed … And you can't be relaxed when you're tense … And so you interestedly proceed ahead … You turn the relaxation control up to a 5 and the tension automatically reduces to a 5 … Now, excited, you continue the process … You turn the relaxation up to a 6 and tension goes down to a 4 … Then to a 7 and a 3 … and so on. You might take them all the way to a 9 and a 1, as a perfect 10-0 might be unrealistic and render you not alert to deal with things needing attention.

This method seems to be very helpful for teaching clients a natural way to decrease levels of tension, stress, and anxiety as described above in my discussion about learning new behaviors that are incompatible with the one you want to change.

With this client, additional time was spent on particular aspects of his psychological problems. For example, he was able to admit that feedback from others determined his feelings of self-worth. As a result, he said he tried not to just win, but "to show up the detractors by winning big." I told him about one of the affirmation cards in Wayne Dyer's book, *The power of intention* (2004): "Other people's opinions of me"(flip to back of card) "are none of my business." However, this did not appear to make much of an impression. One noteworthy statement that came out of an age regression approach was the client's description of how his parents were very critical people and would often say things like: "What is so and so going to think?"

He then suffered an injury, so we never started focusing on his golf game, but he indicated he would like us to do so before he begins to compete again.

Techniques

My standard approach with golfers, after determining their situation, problems, and goals, is to begin hypnosis. In the first session, in addition to gathering some history and learning the client's goals, I use the muscle testing technique (described in Chapter 1) to highlight the importance of the mental aspect of their game. Then I do a test of hypnotic suggestibility. Depending on how much time we have expended on these issues, I may or may not induce hypnosis in the first session. If I do not, I will ascertain when their next competition is and schedule them to return a day or two beforehand.

Once the client is in a hypnotic state (using the induction and deepening techniques described in Chapter 1), I give the following suggestions:

> Dr Bob Rotella is a famous sports psychologist who has written several books about golf. In Tom Kite's foreword to his book, *Golf is not a game of perfect*, he talks about how when he met Doc at the 1984 Doral Open he was in a phase when nothing was going right. He said that Doc merely refreshed his memory about those great thoughts he usually had when he was playing his best and he went out and won the tournament, beating none other than Jack Nicklaus.

> Rotella says that golfing potential depends primarily on a player's attitude, on how well he or she plays with the wedges and the putter, and on how well they think. He tells them to think about their hottest streak, and that the hot streak represents the player's true level of ability. When in it, the golfer is trusting of his or her abilities, playing at their true level not over their head, but at maximum capacity, without self-doubt. He tells them to remember how when in a hot streak "You probably were not thinking about the mechanics of your swing. You weren't getting in your own way from a mental standpoint. You trusted your mechanics."

I tell golfer clients that they are not seeing me to improve their mechanics and that if work needs to be done in this area they should talk to a golf coach. The golfer is then instructed to think about their mental state during hot streaks and replicate that state of mind.

> Rotella says that before taking any shot, you should pick out the smallest possible target, focus on that target and nothing else, and especially pay no attention to the hazards. Know where they are, but focus on your target. If you focus on the hazard, even though it is a negative focus, guess where you are likely to wind up? It is almost like programming in a negative expectancy.
>
> **Pre-shot routine:** A sound pre-shot routine is essential for consistency! If you watch the elite golfers you will notice they all follow a set pre-shot routine. This involves not only physical movement, but also a set of mental thoughts. Some say that this is a major part of the result. It ensures that you set up properly, mentally as well as physically. It helps to block out distractions. And this is what our work together will help you to accomplish. As I said earlier, your golf coach is the one to look to for mechanics. Our work together is to help you concentrate, block out distractions, and focus, using the self-hypnotic techniques I have taught you to accomplish the results you desire. During this state, you assess the shot, pick the club, focus on the target, adjust for the lie and stance variations, and block out everything else. Now visualize the shot, and see the ball going exactly where you choose for it to go.
>
> Next, I am going to teach you a kinetic signaling technique to get you just as relaxed as you are in this chair. As you continue to relax and concentrate in this manner, I want you to touch two fingers together, such as your thumb and index finger or thumb and middle finger ... Good ... This is going to be your ideomotor signal to remind your mind and body to get just as relaxed and to focus just as much as you are right here in this chair. Anytime you are practicing or competing or doing anything that would benefit from increasing your relaxation and focus, I want you to touch two fingers together, and you will get just as relaxed and focused as you are right now, here in this chair. And you can do so throughout your competition, especially during breaks, between shots, and so on.
>
> You might also modify this for immediate pre-shot use. For example, as you relax and focus in this manner, I want you to now imagine your grip on the club just before the shot, how it feels ... And

with that image in mind, associate this current feeling of relaxed focus with the feel of the grip, and when you grip your club before your shot, this will be your signal to get just as relaxed and focused as you are right here in this chair.

Lock it in and flick it out

While out of hypnosis, I instruct the client about locking in good shots and plays and discarding bad ones. For example:

> After a good shot, I want you to lock it in. You might do that clutching movement like Kirk Gibson did when he hit the home run that won the first game of the Baseball World Series in 1988.

While the younger athletes perhaps were not even born then, some of my older clients remember the scene well. For the young ones, I describe the scenario to them, as follows:

> In the 1988 World Series the Los Angeles Dodgers were underdogs to the heavily favored Oakland Athletics, who had won many more games that year. In game one, in the bottom of the ninth inning, the Dodgers were trailing 4-3. After a batter was walked, the injured Kirk Gibson, who could barely walk, was called in as an unlikely pinch hitter. He hit a two-run, walk-off home run and the Dodgers won the game by a score of 5-4. As Gibson was headed to first and as he rounded the bases, he kept making a clutching, pumping motion with his right arm. This precipitated an inspired series which the Dodgers went on to win in five games. *(This approach is similar to what Edgette and Rowan (2003) refer to as "muscle memory.")*

> So I want you, after a good shot, to lock it in. You don't have to be as dramatic as Gibson. Perhaps you might just clench your fist. Just a signal to lock it in … but then forget about it *(I don't use the Sicilian gesture of the hand under the chin when I explain this!)* … You do not want to continue thinking even about a good shot, as it might interfere with preparation for the next … In the case when the shot is less than you are satisfied with, I want you to make a gesture that symbolizes getting rid of it. I learned this from an old spiritual teacher who was teaching us about healing

touch – getting rid of any negativity by shaking out your hand *(I demonstrate the gesture)*. While in competition, you can do this very subtly, if you choose.

World Class Visualizer

Another technique I use with golfers and other athletes is the World Class Visualizer, which I learned and adapted from Mitch Smith (Pulos and Smith, 1998). The client is told:

> I want you to imagine that you have a secret garden … It could be behind your home, or could be somewhere totally different … And I want you to imagine entering that garden, looking around, and then I want you to describe to me everything you see.

Give the client a few minutes, and they will typically describe flowers, trees, perhaps colors and textures, paths through the garden, or a pond. Then I say:

> Very good! Now I want you to imagine that you could put on the head of a world class visualizer … Perhaps that of a famous artist, or an inventor … Einstein was said to have been a world class visualizer … And imagine now that you can see that garden again, but this time through this world class visualizer's eyes and with the benefit of his or her brain … And describe the garden again to me using the world class visualizer's eyes and brain.

Typically, the client describes the garden in much greater detail. For example, they might see not just the flowers, but bees pollinating the flowers; not just the trees, but the texture of the bark; not just the pond, but goldfish swimming in the pond; more and brighter colors, and so forth. Then they are told:

> You have been seeing your golf game for so long through your own eyes and with your own brain. Now I want you to imagine seeing if through the eyes and with the brain of a world class golfer … Someone perhaps that you admire and would like to emulate … Maybe one who is similar enough to you in other ways that you might be able to adopt their techniques to work for you … Someone who knows exactly how to counsel you regarding what

will work for you in terms of your game, from the mechanics of your swing to the mental side of golf … Tell me, do you see, feel, sense, or know anything different from this expert's perspective? *(Give some time to respond)* … Tell me what is different. What comes to you that might be changed to improve your performance? … And now I want you to adopt this perspective or viewpoint as your own … For, after all, it is yours because it came from your own creative mind. Your unconscious mind knows what to do and how to do it!

Space Travel Meditation

Another problem solving technique that can be used in a wide variety of life situations is one I have tabbed "Space Travel Meditation." It is similar to the World Class Visualizer approach in that it is a method of channeling information from the client's own subconscious mind to their conscious mind through an imagined all-wise being. The client is told:

I want you to imagine that you are going to take a trip … And you know, travel can be very educational … People who are well-traveled are often considered to be very wise, and, in fact, that is why schools take students on field trips, so they can be exposed to more of the world and how it works … So I want you to imagine that we are going to take a fantasy trip into outer space.

First, I want you to imagine looking at your home, from ground level, and nod when you have that image in mind … Next, imagine looking down on your home from above, as you might see it from a helicopter or hot air balloon … Things look different looking down from above … If you have ever been on the roof of your home, you remember how things look different from that vantage point … Now you are so high you can see the entire area in which you live, as you might see it from a small plane … And now the whole city as you might see it from a jet plane … Now the entire region of the country, as you might see it from a spaceship or satellite of some sort … Getting higher … You now see the entire continent … and finally the whole of planet Earth … Until you are in outer space … Now I want you to imagine that on your journey you are going to visit somewhere in outer space. It could be another planet, or maybe a star … The only restriction is that it will be only some place that is positive, or at least, neutral … No places that are negative, evil, or scary … And on at least at one of your stops, you are going to meet an all-wise being … He or she or it can be human-like, or it can be very different, but imagine this being has all the wisdom of the universe … All of the wisdom of the cosmos available and this being is willing to share that wisdom with you … So all you need to do is ask the questions, and the answers will come … Most people will ask questions about issues for which they are seeing me. For example: What is this problem blocking me from performing at my highest level? … The next obvious question would then be to ask, What do I need to do differently? … I'm going to remain quiet for a few minutes while you continue your journey, after which time I'll ask if you are ready for me to rejoin you … Then, I'll ask you to talk to me and tell me where you went, who you met, what questions you asked, and what answers came to you.

After three or four minutes, I then rejoin the client and while they are still in a hypnotic state, I ask them to describe the experience. Important insights are often reported from this journey. Later I explain:

We all have much more wisdom, often in our unconscious or sub-conscious mind, than we realize. That is why, for example, when we attend a continuing education conference to learn something new, we might leave thinking, "I knew that!" And the answer is that we often know much more than we realize we know. So this Space Travel Meditation is a technique to channel information from your own unconscious mind, through the all-wise being, back to your conscious mind.

Time continuum-future success technique

After a number of sessions in which the client was given the deepening techniques involving counting backwards, I tell them:

This time, instead of counting backwards, I am going to count forwards and this time I want you to imagine a trip up into the clouds … Perhaps an escalator ride up to a platform in the clouds … Now, this is a fantasy, of course, but fantasies can be very relaxing.

After counting to 10, I say:

> Now imagine a platform in the clouds … White, soft, fleecy, floating clouds all around you … And you are curious about these clouds … You wonder if they will support you … So you experiment … one foot, one leg … And to your pleasant surprise, the cloud does support you … So you step out onto the cloud, sit down or maybe even lie down with your head propped up by one elbow and arm, luxuriating in your white, soft, fleecy, floating cloud … And from that vantage point up in the clouds, you can see the world going on below, people going about their daily routines … And you can even see yourself going through your day's activities … You can also imagine a continuum of time … So that directly beneath you would be the present … But off to the left the past … The near left being the recent past, and the far left being the distant past … *(If investigating possible past events causing self-sabotage, this technique could be a form of age regression, but with athletes, it is often a means of age progression or future projection.)* And off to the right is the future … The near right the near future and the far right the distant future … And we can use this technique to look into the future … Now, we can't predict the future unless of course we are clairvoyant … But we can project how we would like it to be.

From there, the therapist can use the following confidence building method to project future success.

Confidence building technique

Allen (2004) presented a generic script for confidence building in general, which I have modified for confidence building in athletes. The client is told:

> As you now go deeper relaxed … you can begin to realize that with every positive experience, you will grow more and more confident … Increasing your feelings of self-worth, recognizing that more and more you come to realize that only positive thoughts are of any value to you, and negative thoughts can be discarded as having no value … But you also know that an error or mistake, or loss, is only an opportunity to do it differently next time, to improve, to refine … Knowing that even champion athletes are never perfect all of the

time … As the story goes, Thomas Edison was on his thousandth trial of inventing the electric light bulb when a friend commented: "Thomas, I can't believe you don't just give up. I would hate to have to admit that I failed 999 times." To which Thomas reportedly responded: "Oh I haven't failed at all. I have just discovered 999 ways NOT to invent the electric light bulb" … You have all the confidence you need to carry you through your plan to practice until you become better and better, more and more competitive, until you achieve your maximum potential … And only when you have reached your maximum potential, performing to your fullest, greatest potential, might we think about getting even better … Raising the bar, so to speak, to a higher maximum potential … You are calm and relaxed, confident in your ability to learn, to improve, to excel.

Case 5: The child golfer

(This case is presented separately from the prior four because of the inclusion of a telephone consultation.)

The case involves a 10-year-old male golfer with whom I am currently working, so I cannot, of course, discuss him by name. He has been performing fairly well, but his parents were looking for even better concentration and focus. They were concerned especially about how he got so down on himself, filled with self-doubt after he played poorly or even after one bad shot. Since they traveled approximately two and a half hours each way for sessions with me, we decided to always schedule double sessions. I used the techniques described above with him.

The client went to the US Kids Golf World Championship at Pinehurst Resort, North Carolina in August, 2010. We had pre-planned a long distance telephone consult the evening before the competition started but due to his practice schedule and other pre-tournament activities, we were unable to speak until the following evening. He explained that he had shot an 80 the first day and was standing 25th to 30th of 140 golfers. He reported: "I had a good mental game today. I had a new caddie, and he didn't make me get down or anything." He said he was 12 behind the first place entrant and three or four behind number 20. The following script was presented:

> I want you to put yourself into a self-hypnotic state, just as we practice in my office and as you have been practicing at home. Let me know when you are there. *(Client says "Umm.")* Okay, now concentrate on your breathing, slowing it down, just as when you are in a deep sleep ... Now count yourself down from 10 to 1, each number taking you deeper relaxed ... Okay, now concentrate on what I am saying. Tomorrow, you do not need to try to make up the 12 shots to try to be number one. Focus on making up the three or four to be number 20, as was your goal ... And if you happen to be having a great game and think you can do even better, then you can focus on passing more of the leaders.
>
> I want you to practice tonight. Ask mom and dad to go get a cup of coffee while you practice self-hypnosis in the hotel room. Tell them I said to do this. Then I want you to visualize each hole. Each of the 18 holes is the same as you played today, right? *(Answer: "Yes sir".)* So you are more familiar with the course, and you tell yourself: "I've already done this once, so I'll do better this time around." If you had particular trouble with one hole, tell yourself, "Well, I have plenty of room for improvement, so I'll do better." *(Responds: "Yes sir.")* ... Next, visualize each shot before you take it and use the locking in and flicking out technique that we talked about to lock in good and get rid of bad shots. Remember to breathe deeply, just as when you are in the chair in my office, relaxed and *focused* only on that next shot ... Does all that make sense? *(Responds: "Yes sir!")* ... Any questions? ... *(Responds: "No sir!")* ... Great, I am looking forward to seeing you again after you get home.

The parents indicated that they were quite pleased with the results.

In Chapter 6, I present an interview with Brian Kinchen, the subject of Jeffrey Marx's *The long snapper* (2009). This discussion was intended to highlight the unfamiliar mental pressures for some of the more obscure football players (e.g., long snappers, lineman) who are only typically recognized when they make a mistake. However, little did I know how much Brian was involved in golf, so his comments on the mental side of golf are also relevant here.

In summary, a number of different strategies and techniques can be used with golfers. Typically we are not reinventing the wheel, but rather presenting and reinforcing the suggestions given by golf experts such as Rotella (1995, 1996, 2004) who write about techniques to improve golf scores. However, I use hypnosis and self-hypnosis training as a means to reinforce and perhaps even "lock in" these concepts.

Chapter 3

Track and Field Athletes: Sprinters, Distance Runners, and High Jumpers

Whether you think you can or think you can't, you're right!

Henry Ford

"Bannister breaks four-minute mile!" Probably nothing is more indicative of the importance of the mental side of sport than the fact that for so many years a number of so-called experts postulated that humans were physiologically unable to run a mile in less than four minutes. Roger Bannister accomplished this feat in 1954 with a new world record of 3:59.4. The previous record of 4:06.4 had been made in 1937 until a pair of Swedes, Gunder Hagg and Arne Andersson kept lowering each other's records between 1942 and 1945, eventually reaching 4:01.3. Remarkably, shortly after Bannister's feat, his main rival, John Landy, lowered the record to 3:57.9. By the end of the 20th century, Hicham El Guerrouj from Mirocco had lowered the record to 3:43.13. As of November, 2009, the fastest mile ever run was 3:34.45 by Chance Duffy of the United States. Through to February, 2009 the women's world record for the mile run was 4:12.56 set by Svetlana Masterkova of Russia on August 14, 1996. When Bannister set his record in 1954, the fastest women's mile was 4:59.6, so while no woman has broken four minutes and there has been no new record for 13 years, the difference between the men's and women's times is certainly smaller (from 60 seconds in 1954 to 38 seconds in 2009).

Bannister was the inaugural recipient of the *Sports Illustrated* Sportsman of the Year award in January 1955 (1954 Sportsman of the Year). He became quite a celebrity and was the first Chairman of the Sports Council (now Sport England) and was knighted for his service in 1975. After his retirement from running, he also became a highly respected neurologist and conducted some of the early studies on the effects of anabolic steroids on athletes. Some famous and inspiring quotes from Bannister include:

> The man who can drive himself further once the effort gets painful is the man who will win.

> No longer conscious of my movement, I discovered a new unity with nature. I found a new source of power and beauty, a source I never dreamt existed.
>
> Quoted in Cameron (1993)

And my favorite:

> Every morning in Africa, a gazelle wakes up. It knows it must outrun the fastest lion or it will be killed. Every morning in Africa, a lion wakes up. It knows it must run faster than the slowest gazelle, or it will starve. It doesn't matter whether you're a lion or a gazelle—when the sun comes up, you'd better be running.
>
> Quoted in McDougall (2009)

Invisible Barriers

While the importance of "I think I can ... I know I can" philosophy is well demonstrated in the history of the mile run, it is a good example for athletes in all sports. One script that I have used with runners as well as other athletes is Invisible Barriers which I have adapted from Havens and Walters (1989, p. 141). Although I vary the script based on the athlete and his or her particular circumstances, it incorporates the following ideas:

> Have you ever ridden a horse, or do you know anything about horses? *(Most people will respond in the affirmative. If not, you might have to improvise.)* Well, if you ever noticed, sometimes the farmer or rancher will have a fence to keep them in which is electrified ... Not a severe shock, just a mild little jolt to get the horse's attention ... Being pretty smart animals, the horses quickly learn to avoid going too close to that fence ... But then, after a period of time, the electric current can be disconnected, perhaps even

replaced by some ribbon … And the horses will still not touch the fence … An invisible barrier has been conditioned … But then, if one horse were to go through, the others quickly follow in pursuit, without fear … This mental barrier may be much like the myth about men not being able to run a mile in less than four minutes. When Roger Bannister broke the four-minute mile mark, many others followed. It is about the individual's belief system about what he or she can or cannot accomplish.

Another favorite I share with track and field athletes is the story of Steve Prefontaine. "Pre," as he was called, was an Olympic hopeful who was described by his coach, the legendary Bill Bowerman (co-founder of Nike, Inc.), as well as a number of others athletes, as the greatest distance runner in the US. Prefontaine helped inspire the running boom in the 1970s along with contemporaries Frank Shorter and Bill Rodgers. Born and raised in Coos Bay, Oregon, Pre was primarily a long-distance runner who once held the US record in the seven distance track events from the 2,000 meters to the 10,000 meters. He died at the age of 24 in a car accident, before he could vindicate his 1972 Munich Olympics fourth place finish in the 5,000 meters at the 1976 Olympics in Montreal. His training was dedicated to beating Lasse Virén, who won in 1972 and went on to win in 1976. Pre was winning everything in the US and his times were better than Virén's, but he died in May, 1975.

Although his preferred distance in those days was the three mile run, one of his quotes which featured in the movie *Prefontaine* include: "Winning is not about who is the fastest, but who can endure the most pain." Another quote is: "I am going to work so that it's a pure guts race. In the end, if it is, I'm the only one that can win it." And yet another: "To give anything less than your best is to sacrifice the gift." He was inducted into the National Distance Running Hall of Fame.

Case 1: The high jumper

The following case is one that I share with athletes in all sports and which reinforces my philosophy that I do not have to know the sport, skill, or event to generate a successful outcome.

One of the early experiences I had with sports hypnosis, which occurred just after I had returned from an American Society for Clinical Hypnosis (ASCH) workshop presented by Pulos and Smith (1998) was with a young high school high jumper. Her mom called and said that her daughter had been doing fine in both the 200 meter sprints and in the high jump, usually winning both events, but in the last meet did not do well in the high jump. She had started hesitating just before the bar. I informed her that I knew nothing about high jumping, but that if she could get the coach to give me a list of key phrases she tries to instill in her high jumpers, I could reinforce these hypnotically. These included phrases such as "smooth even approach," "lift up off your plant foot," "arch your back," "tuck your butt," and so on.

I saw the client on the evening before a Saturday meet. Hypnosis was elicited using the reverse arm levitation induction described in Chapter 1, followed by deep breathing exercises, and the visual imagery of an elevator ride as the deepening technique. Since I did not expect to see her for more than the one session, I did not spend time talking about the practice effect or the generalization effect as I typically do in the first hypnotic session. (She did, however, come back for a different reason as will be seen in Chapter 4.) I described the relaxing scenes (beach scene and woods scene) with a focus on the key words of *efficiency* and *effortlessness*. I then went through the key phrases provided by her coach while she was in trance. Then, the key words regarding efficiency and especially effortlessness were again introduced with regard to how they would generalize to her approach and jump. I made a recording of the hypnotic session and instructed her to listen to it and go into hypnosis later that evening, again at bedtime, and early in the morning. Finally, she was to practice the three-step self-hypnotic technique I had taught her immediately before her event.

I was invited to attend the meet the next day, and I am pleased that I accepted. Not only did the client not hesitate before the bar, but she jumped several inches higher than she had before. What especially impressed me about this experience is that I had always thought that hypnosis could enable an athlete to achieve their best effort, but not to surpass it. Rotella (1995), for example, talks about helping the golfer to remember his or her best game ever, and to play at that best level. After working with this athlete, however, I came to believe that perhaps some athletes had never yet

performed even close to their optimal level, so their peak performance had not yet been established.

Case 2: *The runner*

I started running in the early 1980s, long before I had developed
an interest in sports psychology or sports hypnosis. I had been a
sprinter in high school, with some attempts at long jumping (to
show how long ago that was, it was called broad jumping back
then), so I was interested in reading as much as I could about distance running. In fact, I was particularly impressed with Jim Fixx's
The complete book of running (1977) and *Jim Fixx's second book of running* (1980). In the latter, he observes that when he wrote the first
book, which was a best-seller, the so-called "running boom" had
not yet occurred. There had been no major emphasis on the physi-
ological and psychological aspects of the sport, and there were few
books on the subject. He notes, however, that in the three years
between these two volumes, millions of Americans had taken up
running for health and pleasure. Fixx describes the effects of running, and by the second volume, even quotes research suggesting
it leads to improved mental functioning. However, although there
is currently a wealth of literature (too many to reference here)
reinforcing the positive effects of exercise on psychological well-
being (e.g., decreased anxiety, improved mood, less depression,
increased energy), much less has been written about the importance of psychology in improving competitive running.

Fixx points out to those who take up running strictly to improve
their fitness that while entering races can help your training motivation, unless you are an elite runner, you should always think of
it as competing against yourself. That is, the goal is to continue to
improve. This is why most runners can quickly tell you their PR
(personal record) or PB (personal best).

I coached marathoners from 2000 to 2005, all of whom signed up
to run a marathon to raise money for leukemia and lymphoma
victims. These runners were typically first timers – although some
had run before in 5k, 10k, and even some half-marathons, none
of them were elite runners. I often recommended Fixx's books to
these athletes, in addition to a number of more recent titles such

as Hal Higdon's *How to train* (1997), Jeff Galloway's *Galloway's book on running* (2002) and *Marathon: you can do it!* (2001), and Michael Sandrock's *Running tough* (2001). *Runner's World Magazine* is also an excellent resource for training tips and articles about improving peak performance. It includes everything from training schedules to nutrition, advice on proper shoes for various types of feet (e.g., normal, under-pronators, over-pronators), stretching techniques pre- and post-race, pre-race meals, and cross-training.

When I work with distance runners in my practice, just as with other athletes, after describing what hypnosis is and what it isn't and discussing their goals, I always use the muscle testing demonstration. This technique serves to reinforce to the client how important mind power is in their pursuit of achieving their goal. I often use the test of visual imagery, and once it is established that they are a good candidate for hypnosis, I begin with the induction approaches and deepening techniques described in Chapter 1. With my non-athlete clients, I often do not start the actual hypnosis until the second meeting, but with athletes, I want to give them a brief introduction to hypnosis in the first session to reinforce their expectancy for success.

Next I discuss the practice effect and the generalization effect and then I proceed with trance ratification. Relaxing scenes are presented (beach and woods), constantly reinforcing the key words of efficiency and effortlessness with an implied idea that this will generalize to their sport, event, or competition. The client is then taught a three-step self-hypnotic technique (see Chapter 1) and told:

> Today our focus was on just introducing you to hypnosis and relaxation techniques, without any specific suggestions about running or competing. Next time, we will focus on specific techniques to improve your performance.

As with golfers, subsequent sessions involve a variety of techniques, including future projection, the World Class Visualizer, Space Travel Meditation, and others. I often introduce these techniques with metaphors or stories about my own experiences with competitive distance running. I had quit running in the 1980s, not to begin again and become competitive until 1997. Therapists might use stories that relate their own experiences. The following are some that I often present:

> Now I know that I am a good hypnotic subject and am suggestible both in and out of hypnosis. When I first started running competitively in my fifties, entering 5k and then 10k races, although gradually but consistently improving, I was never good enough to win a trophy in my age group. The Gulf Coast Running Club gave trophies for first, second, and third place for males and the same for females in each five-year age group. I remember once when I went to Lafayette, Louisiana to visit my daughter and her family and decided to enter a 5k while there that weekend. She took me to the downtown area for the race, and she and my grandson watched at the finish line. Again, I did not place. On the way back to her house, I commented that I guess I was just going to have to find another sport. When she asked why, I responded: "Because I am just so mediocre at running." Her response was: "Daddy, you've never been mediocre at anything you set your mind to." Well, I don't know if that's what did it, but in the next race I entered (another 5k), I won a third place trophy. I continued improving in 5ks and 10ks and occasionally won second or even first place in my age group and in one 5k won the trophy for overall grandmaster (over 55).

Other stories about personal experiences which I believe the runner might relate to are also given. (Note, these stories can be given either in or out of hypnosis, although I typically present them just conversationally.) One such story is as follows:

> I was racing in a 5k race on the Mississippi Coast and wasn't feeling very energetic that morning. There was a female runner in her early twenties that pretty much ran at the same pace as I did, although I beat her to the finish line. Okay, she was a girl, but she was 35 years younger. I always had a good finishing kick – I guess from my early days as a sprinter. This was a hot day and there were not a whole lot of runners entered. As we got into the last half mile or so, the field was fairly spread out. I had her in my sights, but she was considerably ahead of me. I gradually started "reeling her in" as runners often say when they are attempting to pass someone ahead of them. As we got to about less than a quarter mile from the finish, a male friend of hers who had won top overall, came

back out onto the course to encourage her. As he saw me gaining on her, he yelled to her: "Don't let him catch you." She looked over her shoulder and seemed to hit another gear. I remember thinking: "I'm not going to catch her today. I just don't have enough left in the tank." About 1/10th from the finish line, however, my son, who had finished fourth overall, was on the course and he yelled: "Catch her Dad! You can beat her!" Well then it was like I got this burst of energy, kicked into high gear, and caught her just before passing under the clock. I am convinced that without this positive expectancy offered by my son, I would not have done as well that day.

Yet another personal experience which perhaps portrays my competitiveness rather than suggestibility is as follows:

I was running in a 10k race in the late spring and by then it is already quite hot on the Mississippi Gulf Coast. I was running with a younger woman who had become a training partner and was quite an athlete. She was better at pacing and never went out too fast, as I sometimes did. In fact, her pace was often too slow. But we found that by running together, I could speed her up at the beginning and she could help me with my endurance in the later miles of the race. This day we also had a male friend running with us and the three of us pretty much ran together for the first five miles. At the same time, the woman in the earlier story (we were not true rivals since I was competing against males only – but in a way we were) was always close by, either a little ahead or a little behind, but always close. At about five-and-a-half miles, my training partner said: "Okay, Joe, you think you're such a good sprinter, let's see what you've got." I responded: "I don't have anything left. I'm dying here. There won't be any sprinting today." To which she responded: "You big pussy!" At which time I again got that burst of energy and sprinted the last quarter mile. After the race, I saw my rival, and truly not knowing, asked her: "So, did I beat you or you beat me today?" She replied: "I thought I had you today, until J. called you a 'big pussy,' then you took off like a rocket." *(Of course, I do not use the "p" word with young clients.)*

In Chapter 2, I refer to the technique which I call the World Class Visualizer. I had a personal insight experience when I first learned this approach at an ASCH workshop (Pulos and Smith, 1998). At the time, I was almost continually in training for 5k and 10k races, there being some race almost every weekend. I was improving steadily, so in every race it seemed like I was achieving a PR, but still not beating my training partner who was also improving. Typically, at first, she would beat me by 30 seconds or so in the next race. I would beat her time from the last race, but she would have improved as well. In the morning, the speakers had talked about there being a number of different aspects to our lives (e.g., physical, spiritual, social, occupational, sports and fitness). So when they had us practice the World Class Visualizer technique in pairs that afternoon, the instruction was that we could focus on any of these aspects. I remember thinking: "Well, this is a sports hypnosis workshop and I am entered in a 5k race next Saturday, so I might as well focus on that." When my practice partner told me to imagine my sport through my own eyes and with my own brain, I thought about all of the knowledge I had gleaned about running from books and articles. I knew what to do in terms of pacing, negative splits, and so on. Although I had been improving, my PR was still a rather slow 24:15. My goal for the next race was to break 24:00 for the first time. When she told me to see the competition through the eyes of the world class visualizer, I imagined one of the regular writers from *Runner's World* and seeing it through his eyes and with his brain. She asked what I saw differently, and I kept saying, "Nothing, it's all the same as what I know I should be doing." She persisted, however, and finally, she detected a slight change in my expression. She said: "You have something different, don't you?" To which I responded: "I sure do. He said my goal is too low. I should be able to get under 23:00!" The next race I ran a 22:35 – 1:40 faster than my previous best. I often share this story with runners after having had them use the technique themselves. Then, I say:

> This technique is a way of channeling information that is already in your subconscious mind through the world class visualizer's eyes and with his or her brain back to your conscious mind. Subconsciously, we know much more than we realize we know. That is why you may go to a continuing education conference where you thought you would learn something new, but leave saying: "I knew that." Your subconscious often knows much more than your conscious mind realizes … And you can use this technique in other areas of your life … not only this sport or to deal with

new issues in this sport, but in other activities, in relationships, and regarding financial, educational, or vocational issues.

I talk with distance runners about negative self-talk. Many runners tell me that when running an endurance race they have a lot of time in their own head. The runner might think: "What was I thinking? I'm not trained enough to run X (whether it be 10k, half-marathon, full marathon, or longer). I'm never going to finish!" From cognitive behavioral theory there are techniques to circumvent this type of thinking, such as thought stopping and discounting. I tell them:

> When this occurs, you will tell yourself: "I have been training hard for this, and I'm in great shape," or "I'm a fine-tuned machine," or "I'm a tough dude," and so forth, or some combination of these, supplanting the negative thoughts with positive thinking. Your unconscious mind might even come up with its own creative self-statements to reinforce an optimistic outlook for completing the race running strong and fast.

Case 3: The sprinter

At one point in my running career, I was having a number of overuse injuries (torn meniscus, plantar fasciitis, but mostly degenerative issues – remember, I started late) that made training for distance races unwise. I observed that in many of my 5k and 10k races, I would finish with a sprint and be told by the race director at the finish line, "Good kick, Joe." I would typically respond with: "Thanks, I guess I'm basically a sprinter." So I decided to put up or shut up and entered the 100 meter and 200 meter sprints at the Mississippi Senior Olympic Games (for entrants over 50). One of my sisters had coached youth track, and she enrolled one of her friends to work with me on my start; I had not run out of blocks since high school.

I remember training at the New Orleans City Park training track that had been resurfaced a couple of years earlier when the Olympic qualifying meet was held in the city. I met a guy who, although in his early fifties, looked in good enough shape to be a wide receiver for the Saints, or at least a lean tight end. Although we were in different age brackets (I was in my late fifties), and we did not run at the same pace, we would often do warm-up jogs together and talk. He had won in the high jump at the National Senior Olympics and was quite a good sprinter as well. He once watched me training a 100 meter sprint out of blocks, and said: "You'll do alright, Joe. One thing I noticed is that you remember to breathe." He explained that the 100 meter races are over so fast that some runners forget to breathe.

Now, I'm not sure if it was my distance training or my experience with hypnosis that enabled me to "remember to breathe," but shortly before the meet, I asked him a specific question about self-hypnosis in sprinting. This was: "I know with distance running the problem is often negative self-talk. In endurance events there is so much time to think negative thoughts, but also time to replace these thoughts with positive self-talk/affirmations. But in a sprint, the event is over so fast there is not time to think, so how would I use self-hypnosis to improve my time in a sprint?" His response was as follows: "You use the self-hypnosis before the race. Visualize the whole race, from getting out of the blocks to the finish line." So before the race, I found a vacant trainer's table, did a brief self-hypnotic technique, and visualized getting out of the blocks fast, a smooth, easy transition to an upright running posture, and seeing the finish line 10 meters (or yards) past the finish line. This last aspect was to ensure that I maintained a full sprint through the finish line and not ease up before it. In my first sprinting competition since high school, I won the 100 meter sprint and placed second in the 200 meters. My personal experiences and work with other runners has convinced me that the mental side of running is of ultimate importance. Perhaps this is truly what separates the champions from the also-rans.

With all athletes, but especially with those engaged in endurance sports, the poem below, by Dr Carl Touchstone, is very relevant. Dr Touchstone was a highly respected orthodontist from Gulfport, Mississippi, although he lived for a number of years in Laurel, Mississippi. Carl was an ultra-marathoner, including 100 milers, who was said to have run over 150 marathons and 65 ultra-marathons. He didn't start running until age 34 and died of prostate cancer in 2000 at the age of 59. By his own account, he started running in 1974 when he weighed 256 lbs and had high blood pressure (160/100). He had watched his father and brother die from heart attacks at the ages of 53 and 33, respectively. He started off by walking three miles a day for the first six months, then began to jog. Later he started running 5ks, then 10ks, and in 1977 ran his first marathon in a very respectable time of 3:31. This Mississippi boy was well known in the "ultra" circuit nationally and internationally. In fact, there is now an ultra-marathon race named after him which is run in the DeSoto National Forest, just south of Laurel.

He wrote a poem called "Never quit on the uphill." His focus was on how when the going gets tough and one is thinking about quitting, or tempted to at least stop and rest, persistence will be rewarded. The poem, which has implications not only for running and other sports, but for life, concludes:

> Then the crest of the hill comes into full view
> And we reach the top of this problem so new.
>
> Cruising downhill now with strength in our stride
> The wind in our face, with joy and with pride
> "Thank you God for your grace and good will
> To see that we didn't quit on the uphill."

(for complete poem go to
www.ms50.com/CarlT/Uphill.html)

Chapter 4

Gymnastics and Cheerleaders

Don't be afraid of failing because of a mistake;
be afraid of failing to learn from a mistake.

Anonymous

Some might question whether these two topics belong in the same chapter or even if cheerleading is a sport. Despite the controversy, there is no doubt about the athleticism of cheerleaders, so are cheerleaders athletes without an actual sport?

Case 1: The cheerleader

My first experience in this area was with the high jumper discussed in Chapter 3. The client, who had such great success in her high-jump competition after only one hypnotic session and a recorded tape, retired from track and field competition and became a high school cheerleader. Her cheerleading team won many honors, locally and statewide.

When she enrolled as a freshman at Louisiana State University (LSU), she was preparing for tryouts for the university cheerleading squad. Her mother again called me and explained that there was one particular skill, a standing tuck, that her daughter could do just fine if the coach was standing close enough to catch her should she fall, but as soon as he moved away, she would abort the attempt.

Although it had been a couple of years since I had worked with her on the high jump, hypnosis was induced very quickly. Suggestions this time involved primarily mental rehearsal of the standing tuck, using a systematic desensitization approach. First, she was instructed to see herself successfully completing the flip with the coach right there, just as she had done in practice. Gradually, however, the imagery involved him moving further and further away, in a step-by-step fashion, until he was no longer in the picture. I also sent word to suggest to the coach, via the mother, to do exactly that in practices (i.e., move further and further away). A week later, after she did the official tryout, she reported confidently that she had "nailed it!" It was with great pleasure later that year that I watched her on the nationally televised LSU-Alabama football game.

Case 2: The gymnast

The mother of an 11-year-old gymnast called one February, asking if I could be of help. Her daughter had reportedly had a fall the previous May. She had already seen a sports psychologist who was experienced in working with gymnasts and this consultation had proved to have been of some help. However, there were still certain skills on the beam and particular floor exercises that she would not attempt; more specifically, the back layout was her greatest skill difficulty. The gymnast had seen a hypnotist and was given a generic tape (for relaxation and focus), but the problem only got worse.

The gymnast said: "I feel that I could go for it, but then I don't go for it!" She, like the cheerleader above, said: "If the coach stands there, I'll go for it, if not, I won't." She had performed this skill without difficulty before the fall.

Our first hypnotic session involved the reverse arm levitation induction, followed by deep breathing exercises, and the elevator deepening technique. She was instructed regarding the practice effect and the generalization effect, given some tests for trance ratification (with good response), and then relaxing scenes. In these scenes, the focus was on *efficiency* and *effortlessness*. She was told that we would not deal with suggestions specific to her skills until our second hypnotic session, but I wanted her to generalize these ideas regarding efficiency and effortlessness to her gymnastic routines.

In the second hypnotic session, an eye fixation technique was used, followed by the deep breathing exercises and descending a staircase to induce and deepen the hypnotic state. She was then given a modified version of a generic script for sports performance (from Allen, 2004, pp. 325–327). The script involves a great deal of relaxation training, ego strengthening, self-belief suggestions, and visualizing in the mind a successful outcome before making a single move. Allen recommends that clients practice this every day as part of their training. He also reiterates that what happened before is of no value, and encourages clients to focus only on the present moment and the immediate future. He reinforces the idea that the client has all he or she needs to perform at their very best and to believe in themselves as a winner.

Hypnoprojection was then utilized to review performing the skills perfectly in the past (age regression) and then seeing herself doing them perfectly in the future (future projection). These techniques were followed by another generic script (Havens and Walters, 1989, p. 161), involving an approach for rehearsing future performance. While these authors do not mention sports performance explicitly – instead focusing on knowing what to do to achieve your goal – this approach can be easily modified for the requirements of a specific sport. At this juncture, the client was told to ask the coach to move a little further away each day and to practice these techniques at home.

In our third hypnotic session, which was recorded, an eye roll technique was used followed by deep breathing and a flexible approach to deepening (i.e., "As I count down from 10 to 1, use whatever imagery symbolizes for you going deeper and deeper"). In this session, the Havens and Walters (1989, p. 141) script called Invisible Barriers (see Chapter 3) was employed. This script is a metaphor for removing self-imposed obstacles to achievement. There was also discussion of alert trance and instruction in ideo-motor signaling to help her relax and focus during practice and competition. She reported that her mom would not let her compete until she could do "all of her skills," but she was preparing for a meet at LSU in three weeks time.

The following week, the mother reported that her daughter was "cured." She said: "This is the first time in a year that she is willing to go for it without stopping." She added, however, that she hadn't yet had to perform in front of judges! By then it was March, and she observed that they were near the end of the season and if she got to compete it would be in an abridged version, and the next meet would not be until the following September. It is noteworthy that the mother reported that her daughter was listening to her tape every night.

Our fourth hypnotic session involved more future projection plus the World Class Visualizer technique (see Chapter 2). After seeing her secret garden through her own eyes, then through the eyes of a world class visualizer, she was instructed to see her skills routine through her own eyes, then through the eyes of "a world class champion in this sport." (She chose Carly Patterson, who won gold in the All-Around and the silver in the team competition and the balance beam at the 2004 Olympics in Athens.)

After her competition at LSU, the client returned reporting that she had won a fourth place medal on the bars with a score of 9.475, and had scores of 8.925 on the floor, 9.35 on the vault, but fell on the beam, so only received an 8.5. She said that her beam and floor scores were better than before the fall the previous season, but the vault and bars scores were better this year than they were before the injury.

I had asked the mother to obtain some key phrases from the coach used in training his gymnasts. She brought a list which was broken down into the four different events (in parentheses is the client's interpretation, if I asked for one, of what he meant):

- **Vault**: "Punch hard" (hit the board as hard as you can); "block" (use shoulders instead of elbows); "stick it" (which anyone who has ever watched this event in the Olympics knows has to do with the landing and not taking a step).

- **Beam**: "Point toes"; "straight legs"; "slow full turn"; "stretch back walkovers and back handspring" (don't make them short).

- **Floor**: "Control"; "punch up" (go up instead of backwards); "point toes"; "tight body"; "presentation" (form and facial expression; don't look down at floor); "stick it."

- **Bars:** "Belly in, point toes, straight legs, hollow body" (instead of arching); "feet and knees together, jump in hollow" (shape); "stick it."

The ensuing session involved reinforcing these statements hypnotically.

The client stopped coming shortly thereafter, apparently for financial reasons, but this case demonstrated to me just how committed these young athletes are to performing at their highest potential. This 11-year-old, like the other gymnasts on her team, spent every day in training. Her education involved home schooling and seemed to be secondary to gymnastics; the primary focus of her life was preparation for competition.

A follow-up call to her mom one year later revealed that she was no longer competing – she had left the sport in February, 2009. She had overcome her initial fear regarding the fall the previous season, but then some new fears about other skills developed, so they had decided she should quit. I told her that I would have liked to have had a chance to work with her daughter after these new fears developed. She responded: "She is working out on the side now and would like to go back." She said that her daughter's pediatrician had indicated the changes in motivation could be hormonal (she is now 12). I suggested that she might be even more dedicated after the layoff and the realization of how much she missed training and competition. She said that it was all a costly proposition, plus a serious time commitment, and added that the sessions with me were also expensive. She then added: "After she stopped seeing you last year, she continued to improve and did really well in competition." I offered to see her for a reduced fee because she was so motivated and such a pleasure to work with. The mother said they were thinking about letting her get back into serious training.

In summary, these two case examples are but another example of how hypnotic approaches are effective across all sports and that the therapist need not be familiar with the sport prior to working with the athlete.

Chapter 5

Equestrians: Show Jumping

Don't be discouraged by a failure. It can be a positive experience.
Failure is, in a sense, the highway to success, inasmuch as
every discovery of what is false leads us to seek earnestly
after what is true, and every fresh experience points out some
form of error which we shall afterwards carefully avoid.

John Keats

Show jumping, also known as "stadium jumping" or "jumpers,"
is a member of a family of English riding equestrian events that
also includes dressage, eventing, hunters, and equitation. Jumping
classes are commonly seen at horse shows throughout the world,
including the Olympics. Sometimes shows are limited exclusively
to jumpers, sometimes jumper classes are offered in conjunction
with other English-style events, and sometimes show jumping is
but one division of very large, all-breed competitions that include
a wide variety of disciplines. Jumping classes may be governed
by various national horse show sanctioning organizations, such as
the United States Equestrian Federation. However, international
competitions are governed by the rules of the Fédération Équestre
Internationale (FEI).

I had some experience with show jumping in the early 1970s,
when I lived in Memphis, Tennessee. Germantown, just outside of
Memphis, is well known as hunter-jumper territory. At one time,
my former wife, my 12-year-old son and I all took lessons. My wife
sometimes competed in dressage and my son competed in hunter-
jumper classes. He often did well in the 18-and-under division. He
had a good riding instructor, and I, at the time knowing nothing
about sports hypnosis, would attempt to help him focus on the
task at hand. Being a 12-year-old, he enjoyed showing much more
than practicing! I just loved the trail rides in the hills.

Case 1: The show jumper

Years later, I had a client call requesting hypnosis for concentration and focus. It turned out that she was competing in show jumping and felt she was having problems with focusing. In our first session, the approach was similar to that with other athletes. The muscle testing technique was utilized to show her the power of the mind in determining mental and physical strength. Tests of visual imagery suggested that she was a good candidate for hypnotic training and that she was certainly a good visualizer.

Hypnosis was induced using the reverse arm levitation, followed by deep breathing exercises, and the elevator deepening technique. After instructing her regarding the practice effect and the generalization effect, she was given some tests for trance ratification (with good response), and then relaxing scenes. As before, the focus was on *efficiency* and *effortlessness*. She was told that we would not deal with suggestions specific to her competitive riding and jumping skills until our second hypnotic session, but I wanted her to generalize ideas regarding efficiency and effortlessness to her riding and jumping routines.

By the second session, she had already reported feeling much more relaxed and less tense during her practices. This time we focused on future projection regarding her next competition. She was told to imagine riding the course, in her mind, while in this deeply relaxed, hypnotic state. She was also instructed to practice self-hypnosis using the three-step technique (described in Chapter 1). While in a self-hypnotic state, she was directed to mentally rehearse the course and approach to each fence, her horse jumping it *efficiently* and *effortlessly*, and completing the round cleanly and in a good time.

The third session reinforced what we had done the previous week, but with an even keener mental rehearsal of the nuances of the course – the fences, the crowd, and so on. She had a competition shortly thereafter. When she returned to see me, she gushed with joy. She had won her class, but most importantly, she described the changes she had experienced while riding.

She said: "Although my time was excellent, everything seemed to be moving in slow motion. It was like I had so much more time to think. Although aware of the importance of time, I did not feel any need to hurry. When approaching fences I was able to see and recognize the faces of my loved ones in the crowd. This had never been the case in the past. Everything was just so *efficient and effortless.*"

Not long after this I saw another female equestrian, used very similar techniques, and received similar feedback regarding the "slow motion" effect. She also reported everything seeming to function efficiently and effortlessly. The "slow motion" phenomenon is comparable to what I believe happens in other sports, although it is often just written off as "experience." For example, professional football quarterbacks often talk about the game slowing down as they become more experienced. Drew Brees, quarterback of the New Orleans Saints, is famous for his high completion percentage in which he will go through a number of "reads" before finding the open receiver. Running backs also observe this phenomenon when discussing how experience allows them to get better at finding the open hole. Some individuals seem to have an instinct for this, while others talk about experience leading to the game mentally slowing down.

The show jumping coach

Since it had been quite a long time since I had seen these two riders, I was pleased to have the opportunity to meet a former Louisiana State University (LSU) Champion rider who introduced me to her coach, Leaf Boswell, who agreed to an interview. To begin, I showed her the cases above and asked her to give me some feedback and comments on what she thinks is important about the mental side of her sport.

LB: *Oh yes, that is so familiar. That is what we deal with, all of the time. I will talk with a rider when they come out from the course and they don't remember a thing! They'll say: "I remember walking in the ring and I remember walking out." I do have them walk the course and have them then visualize it beforehand, but not in a very concentrated manner. It's more like just walking through and knowing your path.*

But then I do find my riders get better and start remembering. For exam-
ple, they might say: "Yes, I do remember that jump and thinking I need
to slow down a little bit and I kind of just froze up." I know from my
own experiences that whole process, but especially with intercollegiate
competition it's almost a whole new ballgame. I mean I competed from
age 9 until I graduated from high school, then I began to compete inter-
collegiately. And this brings a whole new aspect to it because you have
to ride a horse you have never ridden before. So mentally it is very hard
because you don't know what to expect from your partner, the horse.
At least in typical competition you're riding a horse that you know, so
you are familiar with their little quirks and their responses to different
things, so it is much easier to go in and feel that you know what to expect,
whereas in intercollegiate competition you have no idea what to expect
from this horse.

JT: *So tell me more about that. Who picks what horse a rider will ride?*

LB: *The host school provides the horses and the tack. They have horses*
in different divisions. And all the riders in a class will go to a draw table
and just draw a name.

JT: *Your riders and the host school riders all have to pick?*

LB: *Yes, but there is definitely a home-field advantage because the host*
school riders already know the horses and have practiced on different ones
in their class. They cannot pick their own horse though. If that happens
they will have to put it back and draw again. We do watch the horses in
the morning and make notes about the different animals, and we can talk
to the owners and everyone is very helpful, but still you're getting a horse
you have never ridden before and that usually takes at least a good year to
adjust to. Even riders who are very confident are not as confident as they
would be on their own horse.

JT: *So on the mental side there would be the anxiety about riding a*
strange horse for the first time in competition?

LB: *Yes. Horses are all so different. In our practices I try to make them*
ride a different horse every time to prepare them, and in practice they
will ride the horse a little to practice before actually taking jumps, but
in competition, they go right into the arena and have to start the course
without practicing on that horse. The horse has already been warmed up
by somebody else. So they just get on and go into the ring.

JT: *Wow! So they don't even have a practice round!*

LB: *Right! It is definitely nerve-wracking. I remember when I competed on the team when I was an undergraduate, it was definitely something that took some time to get used to.*

JT: *Are you saying that with experience riders get better at riding strange horses?*

LB: *Yes. It's something they never had to do before college, and they learn to trust in their own ability to get on a strange horse and have confidence in their ability to perform on a horse they have never ridden before.*

JT: *So tell me more about you. How long have you been coaching?*

LB: *I became the head coach of the team in 2006. I joined the team in 2000. At that time we did not have a true coach that was not a rider on the team. One of my friends was acting coach, but I assisted her. Then a lady came in and coached in 2004 and 2005, and I became assistant coach in 2005.*

JT: *Is your team National Collegiate Athletic Association (NCAA) controlled?*

LB: *This is an emerging sport at LSU and we hope that will happen in the future.*

JT: *So the girl that referred me to you is now graduated and coaching?*

LB: *Yes, she is training in Mississippi.*

JT: *Is she pretty good?*

LB: *Yes. She qualified for the Cacchione Cup which was named after Bob Cacchione. She has won a number of competitions and awards.*

JT: *How important do you think the mental side is in show jumping? You know, in all sports, I tell the athlete that the last shot or play or jump, or whatever, is over, and whether it is good or bad, you must now focus on the next move.*

LB: *Yes. One of the big things I tell them in competition is, if they had a bad fence, to move on, recover, and don't let it mess up the rest of their course. It is just one fence and you can still get a good score. You know, they have a number of fences in succession, and if they have one bad fence they have to immediately recover from that and focus on the next one. Move on, or else you're going to have another bad fence because if you take even a split second to say "Oh, that was really bad," then you are two strides into the next fence, so that is definitely an important component.*

JT: *I learned a long time ago to lock in good memories and flick off bad ones, but very rapidly so as to prepare for the next move. Do you do anything with your riders to help them forget the past fence and focus on the next?*

LB: *No, I don't have any kind of physical signal, but I can see how that could be helpful. Of course, their hands are occupied the whole time holding the reins, but I do tell them: land, re-focus, move on!*

JT: *I would imagine that a lot of it is just trying to get them to relax?*

LB: *Yes, especially beginner riders are very tense and trying to hold themselves in a particular position when it should be just a natural response. You know that if you get off and are very sore then you were probably tensing too much. That is one of the trouble-shooting techniques I use. I'll ask the riders where they are sore. I will tell them that when they are tense it will feel bad, and when it feels bad it will make them even more tense. So relaxing is a big thing. One girl just realized that she was curling her toes and it would cause her to tense throughout her legs. So we had to work on that. It is difficult with large classes to get much one-on-one work.*

JT: *One coach I interviewed said she had the most mentally weak team she has ever coached. How do you feel about your team?*

LB: *I have a totally differing spectrum on my team. I have riders that are extremely mentally weak and I have riders that seem not to be bothered by anything and are totally confident all the time. If they have a bad fence, they have a bad fence and get over it. I have no training in working with mental aspects. I have girls that definitely have performance anxiety. They are visibly shaken before they enter the arena – they are shaky, nauseous, and I just do the best I can. For some, just comforting them and telling them everything is going to be okay will work. For others, saying nothing might be best. But I see riders who are so good in practice, but* *then they go to the competition and literally their whole body is shaking. So I definitely have both mentally strong and mentally weak riders, but most fall in-between. There are always more nerves in college competition than when you are just competing for yourself, because of the team. I was always nervous before entering the ring, but as soon as I got into the ring it all went away.*

JT: *I tell athletes that maybe that it is not anxiety at all. It is excitement. You're not afraid. You are ready to get it on – ready to rumble! Anxiety is a type of fear, but you're not afraid of the competition, you're ready to compete. So a little bit of these feelings may be good, or at least not negative.*

LB: *Yes! That is where I was. As soon as the horse's foot touched the floor of the arena, the nerves went away.*

JT: *Did you experience the slowing down described in the case examples?*

LB: *Yes. Not so much like slow motion, but all of a sudden you have time. I would describe it as a slow motion effect, but it is as if once you land you have time to fix the horse's body and do what you have to do to get your best approach to the next fence. I've definitely experienced that and remembering each step, instead of just landing and feeling that you are immediately at the next fence. I try to get the girls to focus on each step. A lot of times they are in a hurry. So I get them to slow down and relax.*

JT: *Are there any books that you get your riders to read about the mental side of competition?*

LB: *No, but I wish there were some. Most of the books are just about equitation, the mechanics – where to place your hands, where your legs and hips should be and things like that. I haven't really read about the mental side. I often tell riders: "rhythm." In other words, do not go too fast or too slow. I think it is a huge part of the sport, and people don't talk about it because they just don't know how. I have some riders that I would love to send to you, if they were able to do that. I could send you that shaking, nauseous girl who is really one of my best riders.*

JT: *That is what I was going to ask. Do you have anyone with all of the physical tools, but needs help with the mental part?*

LB: *Yes, the girl I mentioned is unbelievably talented but still has so much anxiety. I'm bumping her up to open class this year. But she gets to the point before a competition where she will look at me and say: "This isn't even fun!" But it is something she loves to do, and outside of that moment, if you ask if she really means it she will say no. She gets so freaked out. But she is somebody with whom I feel I could have another national Cacchione Cup rider this year.*

JT: *It makes me think that after working with her, I could work with you to help you learn, since there is so little written for equestrians regarding how to better mentally prepare. Just teaching you to employ some relaxation techniques with your athletes might give you the edge over other coaches.*

LB: *That would be great. Because it is something I definitely need to deal with.*

I then showed her the muscle testing approach; she was definitely impressed.

Case 2: The intercollegiate show jumper

Shortly thereafter, the above-mentioned member of Coach Boswell's team did, in fact, call for an appointment. At the first consultation session, she informed me that there was a competition in two weeks time. At the end of the session, when she felt positive about the opportunity of having some "mental coaching," we agreed that I would see her twice a week until she left for the show.

In this session, I asked the typical question regarding how much of her sport she felt was mental. Her response was: "In my opinion, that is my hardest thing." She talked about her friend and former teammate, the girl who referred me to Coach Boswell, whom she said was "so good at that part." On the other hand, she stated: "And I'm a basket case! I start visibly shaking, tear up, get cold sweats, and just freak out."

"With everything?" I asked. She responded: "I'm too nervous to perform, even in school (she is majoring in Animal Science). With my horse, I'm nervous. But I am getting a little better with him."

She noted that the horse is scared too, so she has to learn to be calm for him. She talked about the upcoming meet with their rival school, West Texas State University, and described selecting horses out of a hat as very stressful.

We then did the muscle testing approach (described in Chapter 1) and a test of visual imagery. The results of both procedures suggested she would be a good hypnotic candidate.

First hypnotic session

Before we began the hypnotic induction, she reported how someone had made fun of her after a recent classroom presentation for scratching her arms the whole time. I determined that a lot of work was in order just to teach this client how to relax. A reverse arm levitation induction was utilized, followed by deep breathing exercises, then a deepening technique involving the imagery of an elevator ride. Once relaxed, she was instructed regarding the practice effect and the generalization effect (for improved ego strength), followed by trance ratification techniques. She was told that to get her more deeply relaxed we would use more calming imagery. This involved the beach scene with the key words *efficiency* and *effortlessness*, and the woods scene with the logjam imagery (all of these techniques are described in Chapter 1). When asked what she saw written on the big log, she replied: "relaxed," which she interpreted as her subconscious mind telling her that it was necessary for her to relax in order for things to be unblocked and flow smoothly.

She was then brought out of hypnosis and instructed on the three-step self hypnotic approach (see Chapter 1). I told her to practice several times a day and arranged for her to come back in two days when I would teach her some new techniques.

Second hypnotic session

The client reported that she had practiced but found the techniques hard to do on her own because she kept getting distracted. She reported that it had helped her sleep at night. She added: "I just get so worked up in competition. I'm really stressed, so people can't even talk to me!" She said that when jumping, the jitters go away after she starts, but in flat classes she stays really nervous throughout because there are five or six other people competing in the ring. She added that she is the only one on her team in the open (highest) class, so feels she "has to do it for her team."

It was decided that I would tape this session for her to use at home, but that we would also do a second tape in the next session which would be a shorter version. An eye fixation technique was utilized followed by breathing exercises and then the imagery of descending a staircase. Just as described in earlier chapters, the athlete is told that the use of different techniques each time is by design, so that she can pick and choose which methods she likes best when doing self-hypnosis. Then she was presented with a modified version of Allen's (2004, p. 325) script on improving performance.

Next, she was asked to remember her best ever performance and understand that this is at least her level of performance, but with increased relaxation and focus, she would likely perform at even higher levels in the future. She was told about the movie *For Love of the Game* in which the pitcher (played by Kevin Costner) is able to block out all sounds, almost as if he is deaf, and focus totally on the task at hand. Everything else becomes irrelevant. She was then brought out of hypnosis and instructed again to practice at home (now with the tape).

Third hypnotic session

She informed me that she had practiced at least three to four times a day and had noticed a big difference in being more relaxed. She was given a list of affirmations (see Appendix) and was told to pick out three or four, type them up on her computer in a large font, print them out and place them in various areas around her home where she was sure to look at them often.

As anxiety appeared to be more of an issue with this athlete than with most (i.e., more than just performance jitters), it was decided to do more in-depth work on anxiety reduction. She was taught a modification of the Master Control Room technique (Hammond,

1990, p. 354) described by Tramontana (2009a, pp. 46–47) for decreasing anxiety and creating a natural way to become mellow.

An eye roll induction was used, followed by deep breathing, and she was given an option regarding which deepening imagery she wanted to use. She was then told:

> I remember a ride at Universal Studios where you entered a chamber, like a spaceship. You are strapped in and then propelled into inner, not outer space, inside of the human body. It is an educational ride where you get to see the heart, lungs, and inner workings of the body. I want you to imagine that you can take a trip deep within your own brain. You know, I think of the brain as like a control room ... Which it is ... And I use the analogy of the NASA Space Center in Houston. Just about every space movie involves the astronauts communicating with Houston ... You remember, "Come in Houston!" Well imagine you are inside your own brain, and in this control room there are monitors, switches, gauges, knobs. So you come upon a monitor that is the relaxation monitor ... And just to its left is the anxiety monitor. Beneath each is a control knob ... So to begin, imagine the relaxation monitor reads 1 and the anxiety 9, which might describe the relative anxiety versus relaxation you feel before a competition, or even during it on the flat course ... Then imagine yourself turning the relaxation knob clockwise from a 1 to a 2 with your right hand, and simultaneously with your left hand turning the anxiety knob counterclockwise down to an 8. And this works ... So you eagerly proceed ahead ... You turn the relaxation control up to a 3 and at the same time the anxiety control down to a 7 ... Then, you move relaxation up to 4 and anxiety down to a 6 ... But now, you begin to notice something very interesting. It is as if when you turn up the relaxation knob, the anxiety knob is moving down automatically ... You experiment, and sure enough when you turn relaxation up to a 5, the anxiety knob moves down without your even touching it ... And this is understandable ... Because tension, stress, or anxiety are incompatible responses with relaxation ... what we call mutually exclusive. You can't be anxious when you're relaxed and you can't be relaxed when you're anxious ... So you continue, up to a 6 and a 4 ... a 7 and a 3, 8 and 2 ... Even a 9 on relaxation and 1 on anxiety. With sports performance, we might want to hold on to

just a little tension, just to keep you on your toes and alert … So maybe a 9.5 on relaxation and a 0.5 on anxiety.

After this, she was instructed on the importance of gratitude in sport. For example, she was encouraged to think about how grateful she is for just being able to compete at this level in a sport that she so enjoys. I taught her a prayer that I used to tell my marathon runners, which I had developed years ago from a combination of a book by Wayne Dyer and a tape by Deepak Chopra (both too long ago now to remember exact references). I gave my runners the option of participating in a team prayer, after one of the runners, who happened to be a youth minister, was asked by his teammates to lead them in a prayer before the start of the race. The prayer is as follows:

God, thank you for all of the good things you have in store for me today; And thank you for the courage and strength to handle all of the challenges you have in store for me today *(knowing that there will inevitably be some)*.

I then instructed her, out of trance, on how to use ideomotor signals to remind her to be just as relaxed when performing as she is when in hypnosis (this involved touching her fingers together around the reins in a way that would not affect the horse). We then decided on ways that she could lock in good moves and flick away mistakes (see Chapter 1). The latter involved shrugging her left shoulder very subtly, which she said would be good for her anyway, since she had a habit of dropping her shoulders when things were not going too well.

Fourth hypnotic session

During this session (also taped) the client was given a choice between the three induction techniques she had been taught. She chose the eye roll technique. Once she had closed her eyes, some time was spent with deep breathing. Then she was told:

We have also used different deepening techniques. The first was the elevator image, then the staircase, then in our third session I gave you a choice of either of those, or perhaps an escalator, or gently sloping hill down to a valley or a river. But today, we are going to use yet another approach. This time, I am going to count forwards from 1 to 10, and this time each number will symbolize a higher level of relaxation, 10 being the highest level. And as I count you can imagine perhaps an escalator ride up into the clouds … To a platform up in the clouds. Now this is a fantasy, but you know *(name)* fantasies can be very relaxing … *(Count from 1 to 10 slowly, pacing with her breathing)* … Now, at 10, I want you to imagine a platform up in the clouds … White, soft, fleecy, floating clouds all around you … And you are curious about the clouds … You wonder if they would support you … A few years ago one of the big-name mattress companies had a TV commercial that showed people lying on their mattress and it being "soft as a cloud." So you experiment with one foot, one leg, and to your surprise the cloud does support you … You sit down, perhaps even lie down, maybe with your head propped up by one elbow … Luxuriating in your soft, white, fleecy, floating cloud … And from that lofty vantage point *(name)*, you can look down below and see people going about their daily business. You might even see yourself down there going through your daily activities. But we can also imagine a time continuum … So that directly beneath you is the present time, but off to the left is the past … The near left the recent past and the distant left the distant past … We can also look off to the right into the future … Now we can't necessarily predict the future, unless we're clairvoyant, of course, but we can project how we would like it to be … So first, let us look into the past. I want you to go back to when you first started riding … How old were you?

She said: "10 years old." She was then asked if it was fun and she acknowledged that it was, and also that the first lesson was riding English style. She was instructed:

Keep that image always fresh in your mind. How fun it is and how much you enjoy riding … Now, I want you to go to whatever past competition led you to feel the most self-satisfied you have ever felt in riding. *(She indicated that it was her first time in a jumper class, two summers earlier, and she was on her own horse which was jumping two feet higher than necessary over each fence.)* … Okay, so lock in that memory, and know that the experience that caused the greatest sense of self-satisfaction is just your baseline. From here on you can achieve better and better results.

With the recording equipment off (so the tape would not be too long for her to listen to a number of times before her competitions), she was then presented with the World Class Visualizer technique (see Chapter 1). The primary difference she came up with when viewing her competition through the eyes of a world class visualizer was that her confidence level was much higher.

The client was then given my cell phone number and told to call me each evening after her competition to discuss how things went and anything we may need to focus on. She called me on the Friday evening of the first day of competition (which was on a flat course), and proudly announced: "I did great, Dr T. I didn't shake or cry, or anything. I used the techniques and I got fourth place. I could have done better but the owner told me about how the horse was slow coming out of a turn so when I tried to hurry him he went too fast, costing me some points." I inquired if she had asked her coach if she had noticed a difference, and she responded: "Leaf said: 'Oh my God, it was like a different rider out there.'" She then asked if I wanted to talk to Coach Boswell, and Leaf reiterated how well her rider had done and how she would have won first place if not for the one little error, but how she regrouped very quickly.

Early on Sunday morning the client called me to explain that she had not done well the previous day. In the flat course, the young, nervous horse she was assigned had started bucking, she fell off, and the judges stopped the competition and had her change horses. She said that this pretty much messed up her day, including the jumping classes. I then instructed her to remember everything we had worked on in the office: the deep breathing, use of the ideomotor signaling technique to get just as relaxed as when in the chair in my office, and the techniques for locking in the good and getting rid of any negatives. The whole phone call was probably no more than ten minutes. She said she would practice the techniques during the car ride to the arena. About three hours later I got another call from her. She gleefully announced: "Dr T, I just won a blue ribbon! I used the techniques you taught me and I went out and nailed it!"

Chapter 6

The US Big Three: Football, Baseball, and Basketball

Ability is what you are capable of doing. Motivation determines what you do. Attitude determines how well you do it.

Lou Holtz

Football

Although I have not worked with many football players to date, I certainly have an interest in doing more with football athletes, having played in an independent league in my late teens and early twenties and this being my favorite sport to watch.

Edgette and Rowan (2003) have a section on marketing mistakes in which they discourage sports psychologists from donating time to high school and college teams. They report that although it can be gratifying, it seldom leads to a paid position or many subsequent referrals. While the teams may be grateful, administration never seems to suggest a contract or salary after the initial pro bono services.

I have made attempts to provide my services free of charge (on a trial basis) to the New Orleans Saints on three occasions, all with different head coaches, but never received a response. The first of these occasions was during the Bum Phillips era. He had an All-Pro wide receiver who was reportedly suffering from severe head-aches. There had been no indication of a head injury, so I suspected that it might be stress related. Since I'd had considerable success with hypnosis for reducing headache pain, I offered my services via a letter to the coach. I never received a response. I contacted someone through a mutual acquaintance when Mike Ditka was coach, only to be told: "We already have a sports psychologist who works with our players."

In more recent years, Coach Jim Haslett had a problem with one of his quarterbacks during pre-season and into the beginning of the season. The player was quoted in the local newspaper as saying he was "just having trouble maintaining focus." He told the reporter: "I just wish I had someone to teach me to relax." That sounded like it was right up my alley, so I sent a letter to the coach. After getting no response, I sent word through Buddy DiLiberto, the now deceased but former beloved sportscaster from New Orleans. A friend, who was high up in administration at the radio station where Buddy worked, gave him a copy of the letter to personally hand to the coach during his weekly talk show with him. Still no response! The next summer, I ran into Coach Haslett in a hotel swimming pool on the Mississippi Gulf Coast during the Fourth of July weekend, introduced myself, and told him about how I had been attempting to contact him. He was very gracious and said that he had never received the letter, but that if I sent another, he would certainly read it and respond. I did so, but there was still no reply. I felt that this was too bad for them, because these were all conditions for which hypnosis has proved helpful.

While I may not have worked with many football players, I recently had the good fortune of making the acquaintance of Brian Kinchen and his lovely wife, Lori. Brian was the former professional football player who was the subject of Jeffrey Marx's book *The long snapper* (2009). Brian is from a family of football players who attended Louisiana State University (LSU). His father was Gaynell "Gus" Kinchen, who became something of a folklore figure as a member of Paul Dietzel's "Chinese Bandits". The Bandits, the famous unit made up of defensive second stringers, helped the LSU Tigers go undefeated and number one in the US in 1958. Brian's younger brother, Todd, played wide receiver for the Tigers and then played in the National Football League (NFL) for seven seasons with four different teams. Brian's son, Austin, is now the deep snapper for the Tigers. Brian played tight end for LSU and then played for the Miami Dolphins, Cleveland Browns, Baltimore Ravens, and Carolina Panthers before he was injured. Later, after rehabilitating his knee and hoping to return to the Panthers, he was unceremoniously cut loose. At first, he was optimistic about catching on with another team, but nobody called. As a tight end known for his blocking and tenacity as well as catching passes, he then began practicing to be and later became a long snapper. His idea was that the more skills a football player has the better chance they have of sticking around.

Marx notes that long snappers are very obscure players who, if they do their jobs well, are seldom noticed. He describes how total anonymity is considered perfection for this rare breed of athlete. At the age of 38, after 13 years playing in the NFL and three years away from football, Brian Kinchen was teaching seventh grade bible students. Then, with only weeks left in the 2003 regular season and vying for a playoff spot, the New England Patriots' deep snapper was injured. Scott Pioli, their vice-president of player personnel, had been a personnel assistant when Brian played with the Browns. He called him about coming in for a tryout, along with three other players. Brian got the job, and the rest is history. Brian snapped the ball to Ken Walter, the holder, and Adam Vinatieri kicked the game winning field goal.

What most people do not know is the torment and mental anguish Brian went through in the weeks leading up to that game. These self-doubts continued right up until the kick. Brian, who was always known for having the ultimate in self-confidence, began having self-doubts when he experienced rejections in trying to catch on with other teams. By 2003, he had given up trying and settled into his new lifestyle of teaching in Baton Rouge.

The weeks leading up to the Super Bowl were filled with misgivings. In practice, he began snapping over the holder's head or wide to the punter. He had begun to experience what is sometimes called the "yips" by golfers. The yips are described by Jeffrey Marx, the bestselling author of *Season of life* and 1986 Pulitzer Prize recipient for investigative reporting, as "the inexplicable loss of ability to do something that had always been simple for him." Brian's self-doubt became such a gorilla on his back that he called Pioli four days before the big game and said he wanted out. He told Pioli that he would have to find someone else to snap. After some discussion, Pioli reportedly told him he wasn't going anywhere, he was "in and committed."

Lori Kinchen told me about the trauma on the morning of the game, when Brian called to tell her he had cut his finger with a knife at breakfast. Marx notes that despite struggling in pre-game warm-ups and in the first half, the first field-goal attempt was missed, apparently through no fault of Brian. Later, however, he bounced a snap to the punter. Then, the second field-goal attempt was blocked. Again, Brian's snap was true. But two extra point tries were bounced on the ground, although Walter saved them. He did much better in the second half, however, and Marx observes that just prior to the game-winning kick, "Brian jogged onto the field clinging to the hint of composure he had left. He was basically telling himself to just eliminate everything else – just block out everything else – and get it done" (Marx, 2009, p. 214). This self-talk is what I refer to as a *self-initiated post-hypnotic suggestion*.

Brian was kind enough to agree to an interview for this book. At first, he wasn't sure he wanted his name used, but I explained to him that most viewers, even die-hard football fans as well as young players, have no idea about the psychological demands of this position (long snapper), much less than football in general. I explained to him that to adequately describe this to readers, a personal interview with him would be really helpful.

JT: *Most of our education is learned from the TV announcers, and even though many of them are former players or coaches, they tell us about the pressure on a kicker, especially when the game is on the line. And they educate the public about the opponent trying to ice the kicker. Or they might tell us about how a quarterback, especially the younger ones, might be too pumped up in a big game and throw the ball over the receiver's head. But no one that I know about has ever talked about the pressure on a long snapper before Jeffrey Marx. I think the general fan population has no idea about the trials and tribulations that you guys go through. I know, from talking with Lori, how rough it was for you that Super Bowl week.*

BK: *Yeah, it was! But it was so different. In my regular career, I was always practicing. And I can't compare being in a Super Bowl to when I was playing regularly, because I wasn't. But I can only imagine if I had been in a Super Bowl during my regular playing days, I don't think it would have been as near a big deal as it was when I came back. Granted, when I was playing I was pretty consistent – I didn't really throw bad snaps. My bad snaps were miniscule, as compared to the Super Bowl when they were colossal. Certainly when playing I wasn't that concerned about the consequence of a bad snap.*

JT: *And that is a question I wanted to ask, because you had been away for three years. It is like distance running versus sprints; a sprinter has no time to engage in negative self-talk, while a distance runner has a lot of time. Did you feel that when you came back for the playoff run you had more time for negative self-talk?*

BK: *Oh, yes. When I was playing I was a tight end. That's what I did. I went to meetings and my main focus was on being a tight end. I never really thought much about also being a long snapper. And if that had been what I was doing when I went to the Super Bowl, it might have been the same. But when I was signed to just be the snapper for punts and field goals, it was different.*

JT: *And after three years away.*

BK: *Right! If it had been during my regular career, I would not have been thinking about a bad snap maybe losing the game. I mean, I wouldn't have wanted to throw a bad one, but it wouldn't have been such an issue. But putting me in a position where I was just a long snapper was new. I had never done that before. I had never just sat on the sideline and gone in to snap for a kick. I didn't even like those guys! It was very unique for me.*

JT: *So you had more time to think?*

BK: *Oh, yeah. I was around a lot of guys I didn't know. Then throwing a bad snap in that first game against the Titans, it creates this seed of doubt. Then during Super Bowl week, when I threw that bad snap, that colossal bad snap, this started to chip away at my brain.*

JT: *This was in the game or in practice?*

BK: *In practice. The first practice before the Super Bowl, I threw the same bad snap I threw in the Titans game. I tried to throw it too fast, and when you do that it is usually short. And I felt I couldn't relax and concentrate, if you will. It was just like I mentally threw up. My anxiety was fueled by the fact that you knew, if it was a defensive struggle – the Panthers had a very strong defense and so did we – that there would be very little scoring, and I knew it could come down to a field goal. And that kind of hung over me the whole time, because it was such a strong possibility.*

JT: *Now there was a time during that last week when you wanted to come home?*

BK: *Yeah!*

JT: *And what changed your mind besides Scott Pioli?*

BK: *Well, I knew Scott well enough to know that he would talk me out of it. And I knew I would have future regrets. Maybe I just wanted to hear myself say it. Realistically, I probably would have been very upset if they had replaced me with somebody else.*

JT: *Were you down on yourself?*

BK: *Yeah, I can get into self-pity. But realistically, I know I just did not want to be the reason they lost that football game.*

JT: *I read something recently about Pete Carrol saying that when he was in graduate school, he read the book* The inner game of tennis *and learned the importance of quieting the mind to increase focus and concentration. Did you have any such experiences?*

BK: *I am just who I am. And I just learned not to think about it. Not to think about anything.*

JT: *So what was your thinking when you were going in for that game winning field goal?*

BK: *I was just comfortable with whatever the outcome. I had submitted to whatever happened, happened! And the main thought was not to be tentative. I remember Trey Junkin doing that and he botched the snap two years earlier. He was so tentative. And I didn't want to do that. I thought, if I'm going to screw it up its going to be a rifle shot, nothing tentative. I'm going to throw just like I always throw it. Just release to the target. Just relax and do what I do. I had been snapping balls since I was 16 years old. I had done it thousands of times. Just rely on what I knew I could do – and know I'd be alright.*

Brian seemed to then digress slightly to talking about a golfer he watched recently who was so nervous he blew the lead on the last hole. He added that he had been at the tournament, playing for money. Then he came back on target by saying:

BK: *And I see snapping as being just like golf – moving a stationary target. It's different than catching the winning touchdown pass when* *playing tight end. In those cases, the adrenalin is flowing and the ball would come and I'd just make the play. Not think through it, but just rely on what your body is already trained to do. But when you have a stationary object, it's different.*

JT: *I didn't realize that you had played golf competitively, and you know they often say golf is so much more of a mental than a physical game. So do you think being the long snapper in a championship game is more of a mental thing?*

BK: *Well, there is one tournament, an individual stroke tournament, I played in for 12 years that is for prize money. In the year of that Super Bowl in February, 2003, I played in that golf tournament in mid-April. And I hadn't been playing much golf before then. The first day I was 5 under – I shot 66 and it was a par 71. I had won it in 1997 with a shot that was on the golf channel – it was a big deal.*

After he described a number of details about his performance, Brian talked about his final shot on the last hole. He was feeling a great deal of pressure and was really nervous.

BK: *I thought, I've just snapped the ball for the winning field goal in front of millions of people on the biggest stage there is in football! This putt is nothing compared to that!*

JT: *That's great. You reframed it to reinforce your own self-confidence and take the pressure off.*

BK: *I just drained it – knocked it in the back of the hole. I won the tournament and a nice prize check. I've thought about that moment a lot, and talked about it in my acceptance speech.*

JT: *Your statement to yourself: "This is nothing, I snapped for the winning field goal in the Super Bowl" reminds me of Tony Robbins' tape on motivation. He talks about the young basketball star who had been having the worst night in his career, but wanted the ball for the clutch shot and won the game at the buzzer. When interviewed later about why he wanted the ball after going 0 for 13, he said: "Well, I'm a 55 percent shooter. I figured after missing that many, my odds were way up!" Is that kind of what you did on that snap – think, well, this is just what I do?*

BK: *Oh, yes. My memory is really foggy about that snap and kick. It was like I just shut everything down. I knew eventually it would just be over, and all I wanted to do is what I had always done. And I did. I threw a perfect ball. You couldn't ask for a better snap.*

JT: *So do you think you went into an automatic trance?*

BK: *Yes, I just thought about nothing and waited for the holder's hands.*

Brian then proceeded to talk at some length about golf competition. He currently works as a high school football coach but his passion for golf and for competing is obvious. I surmised that this is likely true for athletes in many sports who perhaps become too old to perform at a high enough level to compete with younger stud athletes in the more active physical sports such as football, basketball, track, and so on, but can still compete quite well in the more mental game of golf for quite a long time.

There are many inspirational movies about football teams and players, and a number of excellent quotes from players and coaches, such as Vince Lombardi. A good example is from Joe Namath, who predicted that his New York Jets would beat the Baltimore Colts in Super Bowl III. The Jets were the underdog that day, and in the two prior Super Bowls since the NFL and American Football League (AFL) had merged, no AFL team had won. Namath is quoted as saying: "See your future, be your future!" What an excellent example of future projection. These examples can be used with players, as well as discussing more specific instances of the importance of mental preparation. I tell athletes in all sports, while talking about visualizing success:

> When Morten Andersen kicked for the New Orleans Saints, you could watch him go through a pre-kick ritual. And I don't remember if he kicked some balls into the net first or got on one knee and put his forehead in his hand first, I know he did both, but I've been told that when he put his forehead in his hand, he was visualizing the ball going through the uprights. I'll bet he wasn't thinking about wide right or wide left, because if he did he would be mentally programming failure, not success.

Case 1: The high school football player

One recent experience I had involved a 16-year-old who was initially referred to me for an attention deficit hyperactivity disorder (ADHD) evaluation. After the testing showed signs of ADHD, his primary care physician prescribed a Daytrana (methylphenidate) patch. In addition, however, I told the parents that counseling might also help, and that I could perhaps teach the client self-hypnosis to help control his impulsivity.

Once we got into the hypnotic training, he asked me if hypnosis worked for sports. He played linebacker and was the punter on his high school junior varsity football team. He said he sat on the sideline for varsity games, but rarely got to play in those games. I informed him that I certainly did use hypnosis to improve sports performance and, in fact, that working with athletes is one of my favorite things to do. When he returned after the first session – in which I did some basic, introductory hypnotic work, taught him self-hypnosis, and spent some time teaching him visualization techniques – his father, who was in the waiting room, said to me, "I don't know what you did last week, but he had the game of his life!" In the next session, the client reported, "I used visualization and it worked!"

At that time, the season was ending, and we are both looking forward to further work on improving his athletic performance. In a recent follow-up appointment he said that he continues to practice self-hypnosis and added: "When I do it at bedtime, I can feel my own pulse and it helps me sleep at night." He also said that his team was in spring practice and he had noticed improvement in his punting, noting that he is much more focused on the mechanics of his drop, the contact with the ball, and so on.

Pete Carrol, until recently the Head Football Coach at the University of Southern California (USC) (now with the Seattle Seahawks of the NFL), wrote a foreword to the 1997 paperback edition of Timothy Gallwey's *The inner game of tennis*. He says that when in graduate school, years before, he had read the earlier edition and learned about the importance of mental quieting techniques to help focus and concentration. He describes how the 2005 National Championship Game was a great stage for his USC Trojans. Billed as the "Game of the Century," USC was the top-ranked team and played the second-ranked Oklahoma Sooners in the nationally televised FedEx Orange Bowl in front of a record audience. He notes that while the game would be highlighted by athletic prowess and memorable playmaking, a more subtle battle would be waged in the minds of those same players. The mental aspects contributing to this great physical performance would be crucial to the outcome: "Tim Gallwey has referred to these mental factors as 'The Inner Game.' Coaches and athletes alike must clear their minds of all confusion and earn the ability to let them play freely."

Baseball

In Morgan's (2002) chapter on hypnosis in sport and exercise psychology, he references a report by Johnson (1961) regarding successful use of hypnosis with a professional baseball player who was in a batting slump. A typical 300+ hitter, he had not had a hit in the last 20 at-bats. Neither he nor his coaches could figure out if there had been a change in his swing, stance, or something else. In hypnosis, the player was able to achieve the proverbial "flash of insight" allowing him to become aware of specific problems with his swing that he was unaware of consciously. He went on to finish the season with a much higher average than he'd had before the slump began.

Coach and athletic director, Mike Marshall (2001) wrote an article about the mental side of pitching. Dr Marshall is a former Cy Young award pitcher (1974, with the Los Angeles Dodgers) who played 14 seasons with nine different teams, from 1967 to 1981. He was able to continue his education while playing and received a doctorate in Exercise Physiology in 1970. He observes:

> Pitchers have to develop an intuition about the hitters. If they can't develop it by feel, they have to do it by design: keep track of what pitches they throw and what the hitters do against them. In short, keep pitch records and keep looking at the videos and films. That is critically important. It will help them get an intuitive sense of what the hitter is thinking and doing. I used to look the hitter right in the face, and I could sense what he was looking for, and I'd never throw that pitch.

I remember going to the 1975 All-Star game and running into Dave Concepcion, the great Big Red Machine shortstop. Dave asked me if I was a mind reader. I said no, what do you mean? He said: "Whatever pitch I'm looking for, you never throw."

This reveals how with pitchers, the mental side of the game is two-fold. They must think about how to approach a certain batter, while also being calm, relaxed, and focused on their own mechanics.

There are some good inspirational movies about baseball. I often talk to athletes about the movie *For Love of the Game*, in which Kevin Costner plays the star pitcher in the twilight of his career. I ask them to notice what he does to block out distraction, especially when playing in the opponent's ballpark. The home crowd is typically very hostile. They heckle him and tell him what a bum he is, and so on. His ritual is to say to himself, "Clear the mechanism," and it was if he suddenly becomes deaf, blocking out all sound. This approach is a form of self-hypnotic trance induction. Sometimes it helps with athletes in a variety of sports to be able to achieve a type of tunnel vision. In this way, they focus solely on the goal response, blocking out all distractions.

Case 2: The baseball pitcher

I worked with a young pitcher with the local Triple A team, the New Orleans Zephyrs, who complained about difficulty maintaining focus. The session incorporated a reverse arm levitation induction, followed by deep breathing exercises, then the visual imagery of descending in an elevator from the tenth floor to the first floor. After discussing the practice effect and generalization effect (see Chapter 1), followed by trance ratification, it was obvious that he was in a deep hypnotic state. He was given relaxing scenes and the logjam imagery was used to determine if there might be a particular factor blocking him from focusing. What he saw written on the log was, not surprisingly, "concentration."

The following post-hypnotic suggestions were given:

> You told me earlier that you had seen the Kevin Costner movie, *For Love of the Game*. Remember how he uses his special words,

"Clear the mechanism" to block out crowd noise and focus totally and completely on the next pitch … Well, I want you to do something similar to create a kind of tunnel vision such that you are able to block out all distractions, both in the ballpark and away from it, whether personal or professional, and focus all of your mental energy on that next pitch … When the pitch turns out the way you planned for it to, which I expect will happen the majority of the time, you might lock it into your muscle memory by very subtly clenching the fist of your throwing hand. If, however, the pitch is not as you would like it to be, do a quick, subtle flick of the fingers on that hand to symbolically get rid of the memory.

He returned the next week reporting improved focus. In our second session, we used the imagery of the World Class Visualizer (see Chapter 2) in addition to reinforcing what we had done in the first session. Although a third meeting was planned for him after the next road trip, he cancelled that appointment saying that he had been called up to the "Bigs," as they call it in baseball (i.e., Big Leagues), so we could not continue our sessions.

Basketball

Although I have not yet worked personally with any basketball players, I often tell athletes in other sports the following story which is presented in greater detail than it was earlier in the chapter when I briefly mentioned it to Brian Kinchen:

In Tony Robbins' audiobook *Unlimited power* he talks about many people who have overcome great adversity. These individuals often persevered through many failure experiences and finally succeeded. One of his stories is about a basketball player who was the star of his team but having a terrible game. The game was very close and it became crunch time – one more shot to take before game's end. If the shot was made, the team won, if missed they lost. In the final timeout, the coach asked: "Who wants to take the final shot?" (I believe he should have said: "Who wants to make the winning shot?"). The star, however, who had been having such a terrible night shooting, volunteered. Coach asked: "Are you sure?" He said: "Get me the ball. I'll make the shot." Which he did, and his team won. Later, a reporter interviewed him about getting the ball for the clutch shot. He asked: "After missing so many shots tonight, what made you think you could make this important shot at crunch time?" The player responded: "Well. I am a 55 percent shooter. After missing 13 in a row, I figured the odds were in my favor to make one."

This story again reinforces the importance of positive thinking. As Wayne Dyer describes in *The power of intention* (2004), affirmative thinking and imagining success (which hypnotherapists refer to as "future projection" or "age progression") is extremely important in achieving success, regardless of the venture.

Another technique for achieving positive outcomes is one I learned from neurolinguistic programming (Bandler, 1982). After trance induction, this method involves the following suggestions:

I want you to imagine sitting in a safe comfortable room and watching a wide-screen TV that has a picture-in-picture component. I call this a "split-screen" approach. So I want you to imagine the picture on the screen showing how you have been performing your event in the past, in the manner that you feel needs improvement … Now, in a tiny insert in the lower right hand corner, you see yourself performing at your best possible level … And then we are going to go through a fading process in which the big picture becomes smaller and smaller and dimmer and dimmer … The little picture, the way you want things to be, becomes larger and larger, brighter and brighter. About halfway through this fading process the screen will be half and half … But you continue … It is as if the new picture, the way you want things to be, is pushing the old image off of the screen … Until all you have left of the old picture is a small, dim image of the way things used to be … Notice we do not get rid of the old image completely … It is as if you are going to put it on a shelf in the back of your mind … Just as a reminder of how you don't want things to be … And you really embrace this new image of how things are going to be. *(I typically have them repeat this process three times, which I tell them is the magic number to lock this image into their subconscious.)*

In summary, these three sports are the ones of greatest viewing interest in the US, especially at the professional level, with big TV contracts and large player salaries. However, most casual viewers, as well as high school and other aspiring players, have no idea about the depth of the mental side of these sports. It was not until I finished reading Sean Payton and Ellis Henican's *Home team* (2010), that I realized the full mental dimension of the on-sides kick that the New Orleans Saints recovered on the second-half kickoff of the 2010 Super Bowl. For example, the Saints had the option as to which side to defend in the second half. The side Payton chose meant that the ambush on-sides kick to the left would have put the ball right near the Indianapolis Colts bench. As the coach explained, if there was a scrum for the ball – resulting in a human judgment call – who would get the ball? You never want that decision to have to be made around all of the blue jerseys, the coaching staff, and everyone else from the Colts' bench. So he quickly changed his plan and told the official he wanted to kick right to left, not left to right. The Saints recovered and succeeded in this unconventional move so early in the game. They went on to score and basically took the momentum away from the Colts.

Chapter 7

Softball (Fast Pitch)

I'm a strong believer in luck and I find
the harder I work, the more of it I have.

Thomas Jefferson

Women's softball (often referred to as fast pitch, as opposed to the more traditional slow pitch game) is a very popular sport at the intercollegiate and Olympic level. At the 2004 Olympics, in Athens, the US Women's National Team was anointed as the "Real Dream Team" by *Sports Illustrated* and their performance has gone down in history. The squad, coached by Mike Candrea, was considered the best women's softball team ever assembled and possibly the most dominant Olympic team of any sport. With its perfect 9-0 record and its string of eight consecutive shutouts, the team proved it was indeed something special. The US outscored its opponents 51-1 in nine games and did not allow a run until the sixth inning of its final game.

As I had not previously worked with a softball athlete, I wrote to the women's softball coach at Louisiana State University (LSU), Yvette Girouard, requesting an interview with her to learn more about the mental side of the sport, from a coach's perspective. In her reply, she observed that she got my letter just after the father of one of her players mentioned that one of the pitchers might benefit from hypnosis to help her focus. She added that this girl had a lot of anxiety, but she hoped to send two pitchers to me, so it would not look like she was singling out the one with concentration problems.

JT: *Yvette, as I explained briefly in our phone conversation, my basic premise is that the therapist does not need to have played a particular sport or even to have worked with athletes in that sport to be effective when working with a new referral as long as the therapist can get some feedback from the athlete, or parent if a young athlete, or directly from the*

player's coaches regarding what are the key mental concepts they are try-
ing to instill in their athletes. Although I have competed in various sports,
I don't have to be an expert in the sport, but rather an expert in teaching
concentration and focus. I tell the athlete, "I'm not going to teach you the
mechanics of your sport – that is the coach's job – rather, I am going to
teach you to focus, to concentrate, so that you can perform at your peak
level."

I then told her about some examples of cases in which I had
solicited information from the coaches, such as the high jumper
(Chapter 3) and the gymnast (Chapter 4). I also told her about my
experience in the first sports hypnosis workshop I attended; Mitch
Smith had talked about how he could never break the top ten in
racquetball before he learned hypnosis and self-hypnosis and how
after he was the world champion seniors player several years in a
row. I explained how he instructed the workshop participants to
lock in a good shot by clenching the fist into memory. And how
when I asked him what he did after a bad shot – like why not
shake it off with a motion of the hand to symbolize getting rid of
the memory – he said he might try it. I added how I used this with
a University of New Orleans varsity volleyball player (see Chapter
9), and watched her in a game using these ideomotor signals to lock
in good plays and get rid of bad ones. But the idea was to not dwell
on either good or bad but to attend to the next play or shot. I also
explained how I tell athletes about Tony Robbins' example of the
basketball player who was having such a bad night but drilled the
winning shot at "crunch time" and how important self-confidence
is in competition. I shared with her some of the material discussed
in Chapter 2 about how with golfers I use many of Rotella's suggestions which he gives conversationally but I give hypnotically.

YG: *So you tell them these things while they are under hypnosis?*

JT: *Yes, and I also work with them on blocks – what mental thoughts*
might be blocking them from performing at peak level.

YG: *This kid that I mentioned on the phone that I might want to refer*
to you stays angry all of the time. It is like she needs some kind of anger
management. She sees our sports psychologist and she sees a psychologist
at home, but it hasn't helped. And she is going to have a sad career – she
could have had such a good career but she gets in her own way.

JT: *There have been times when I have approached teams about working with athletes who were struggling, and they would say something like, well, we already have a sports psychologist. And I say, but this is a little different from the approach that most psychologists use.*

YG: *And this young lady would have to do it on her own. I approached our compliance officer, and we couldn't pay for it – her parents would have to – because she would have to do it for her own self-improvement. I'd like to use every avenue there is to help her because she has such potential. So how many sessions does it take before you start seeing results?*

JT: *It depends. One of the college golfers I have worked with, who interestingly had had some sessions with Rotella, reported to me that he shot his best game ever after one session with me. Others might take several sessions to really learn to use the techniques, then might come back before important competitions. It's not usually long term, unless we are dealing with a lot of other stuff.*

YG: *Yeah. Maybe some other stuff that is going to manifest itself. I would've never even considered it. But the dad of the number one pitcher said about the number two pitcher, "We need for her to be good for the whole team's sake. You know, maybe she needs to go see a hypnotist." Then, shortly after that discussion, I got your letter about wanting to interview me for this book. Otherwise, I would not have even known about you.*

She then asked me if I do hypnosis with problems such as smoking.

JT: *I work with smoking cessation regularly, and with good success. But one of my favorite things is working with athletes, because they are so highly motivated.*

YG: *Exactly, they want to succeed!*

JT: *And they are used to repetition. When I tell an addict to practice self-hypnosis X number of times a day, they usually don't. But athletes are so used to repetition that you can tell them to practice many more times per day and they do it.*

YG: *Right! They'll do it.*

JT: *I'd like to hear more about how you see the mental side of softball. You mentioned to me about pitchers who ask: Why can I do it in the bullpen but not in the game?*

YG: *We do some mental exercises. We have them listen to CDs. We have packets of mental exercises and have a lot of sports videos we have them watch before the games – motivational videos.*

JT: *One of the ones I recommend to athletes in all sports is the baseball movie* For Love of the Game, *with Kevin Costner, in which he is a pitcher who blocks out noise by telling himself: "Clear the mechanism." It is a trance state he is putting himself into to cause deafness to attempted distractions from the other team's fans.*

YG: *Right! We make our own – we take clips of* Gladiator *– so the idea is that whatever comes out here we stay together. We do different ones for every series. We do a lot of stuff, although sometimes it doesn't seem like it is working.*

JT: *But that's great. It is putting positive suggestions in their minds.*

YG: *It is all positive, all pump-up stuff. We also tell them to find a focal point on a field and if they start to stress out to look at that one point and ignore everything else for a moment – sort of like your clench-and-release thing.*

JT: *One of the things I do with athletes is to teach them ideomotor signaling. For example, I tell them while they are in a deeply relaxed state to touch their thumb and index finger together and that is their cue to get just as relaxed as they are right here in my chair. So any time you are in an activity and you start feeling stress, anxiety, or worry, just touch that thumb and index finger together and, I repeat, that is your signal to get just as relaxed as you are right here in this chair.*

YG: *So you interview them and then decide which course to take? And how long are they in hypnosis?*

JT: *Yes, and the first time I actually do hypnosis is during the second session with the client. I like to have at least the full 45 minutes the first time to orient the client as to what we are doing and why. Later sessions involve shorter and shorter induction times.*

YG: *I'm sure you've been asked this before, but have you ever not been able to get anybody out after you have put them under?*

JT: *No, because they are not in an unconscious state. It is like the body is asleep but the mind is alert. I often tell clients: "If I were to walk out of the room for some reason and a truck ran through the building and crushed me, you would come out to see what all the noise was about."*

YG: *Now, if this girl was to come in and her mother wanted to come in with her, would you have any problem with that?*

JT: *No, and remember, I sometimes work with very young clients, so to make both the client and parent feel more secure, I tell the parent: "If you feel better about being in the room, that's okay as long as you do not try to help – that would be too distracting to your child and to me." Most often, if the parent does want to be in the room or if the child wants the parent present, that is only for the first session, after which they have a better understanding of the process and are no longer fearful of it.*

YG: *Good, because you know some people might be naturally skeptical at first.*

JT: *I usually discourage it in the second session, especially if the athlete is having some kind of mental block and we attempt to investigate. I might tell her to imagine watching a movie about herself, and we are going to rewind the film to some significant event in her past that is causing the present problem. Well, it might be something she does not want her mother to know about, especially if the mother is somehow involved in the causation of the block. That is why I give a very detailed orientation as to what hypnosis is and what it is not.*

YG: *Yes, we know these kids are talented. That is why we recruited them. But we don't know these things until we turn the lights on, and we see that despite all of the talent, they simply cannot perform.*

JT: *I usually use this demonstration with all athletes and with parents present if a young athlete. Let me show you if you will. I did this with Tony Minnis and he said: "That's amazing."*

I then demonstrated the muscle testing technique (described in Chapter 1), with the expected result.

YG: *So how long have you been a hypnotist?*

JT: *Since 1978, but remember, I am a psychologist first, licensed in 1971, and have certification in clinical hypnosis, and just happen to have a special interest in applying these techniques in sports.*

YG: *Okay. I'm definitely going to present this to the player I told you about and see if she is willing. And the other pitcher's father said we could have you see her, as well, so it did not look like we were singling out one player we thought had problems.*

JT: *Well, I'd like to work with her, with both of them.*

YG: *Everything she does is tense, and she has had some arm injuries because of that. Everything is all out. She had to make straight A's. She's driven, but just doesn't know how to relax.*

JT: *But you know, sometimes people like that are just as driven about learning these techniques. They jump in with both feet and say they are going to learn this, and they do!*

YG: *This kid could potentially be an All-American. She is her own worst enemy. I really want her to come to see you. If I were allowed to pay for it myself, I would. But I think especially if her parents can come, they might do it.*

I have talked with Coach Girouard on a couple of occasions since then and I expect that if not the one she was referring to, some other softball players will be referred in the future.

Chapter 8

Tennis

You have to have the desire to achieve, to do better
and do more and continually do, do, do. It's an
insatiable desire to not only win, but not to lose.

Serena Williams

I had not previously worked with a tennis player at any level,
although I hoped to do so in the near future. However, Coach Tony
Minnis, the women's tennis coach at Louisiana State University
(LSU), was gracious enough to grant me an interview for this book.
He also coaches the Southern 18s (high school seniors, juniors,
and sophomores who are prospects to play at the college level)
in the National Team Competition sponsored by the US Tennis
Association. Since the interview, I have worked with one of his
varsity players; the case example follows the interview below.

JT: *One of the major premises of the book is that I don't have to have had
experience working with athletes or playing certain sports, as long as I
have some input about what are the key mental concepts his or her coach
is trying to instill. Since I have not worked with a tennis player, I thought
you might be a great resource to help me understand the mental side of
tennis. When we talked briefly on the phone yesterday, you seemed to be
very deeply into the mental side of tennis.*

TM: *Well, I think tennis is the quintessential sport that involves the mental side, similar to golf, but even more so. As a coach for 19 years and as
an athlete – I played at a high college level – the consistency I have seen
in kids that succeed is between the ears.*

JT: *Between the ears?*

TM: *Yes, I tell people all the time that when I recruit for tennis, I look at
results. You can have a kid who is slow, not as gifted as some others, but
if they are really tough up here (points to head), that's what I want. You*

can have a kid who is 20th in the country and another who is 60th, but evaluating and recruiting for tennis is different from football, because in tennis it's head-to-head competition. I think that my team for next year has the physical tools, but do we have the mental toughness to get us there? It's a sport where there is no substitution. When you're out there, you're out there. So if you read much about tennis, you will read estimates that tennis is about 85 to 90 percent mental.

JT: *You described tennis as "the ultimate individual sport." I was thinking in terms of tennis being a fast-moving sport. Like with running, there is a big difference between sprinting and distance running. Sprinters have little or no time for negative self-talk, whereas distance runners have lots of time for that. I thought tennis was so fast moving, but you said something on the phone about 20 to 25 seconds between serves?*

TM: *Oh, it would blow your mind. In tennis, more that any sport, there is no doubt that there is more negativity that goes on up top. I talk about this over and over. I videotape my players to show them the body language they show after a bad shot. It is so obvious they get down on themselves. Take John McEnroe – you get kids who buy into that negativity. They get caught up in it. Getting frustrated and letting their emotions flow. I have rules like you can't throw your racket. When you're playing tennis, you have 25 seconds after a point to the next serve. So we're talking about keeping focused so you don't get caught up in the negativity. You would be shocked if you came to a match or a practice and just observed the body language. It's hard to see it on TV because of the cameras. But even the pros, if you watch them close up, you will see them get down on themselves. In an average match, you probably play 140 points, and during that time, maybe you win two and lose one, lose one then win two – it is up and down and up and down. And for the coach, when the negativity kicks in and you lose several points in a row, probably the comment I've made most in my career is "Let it go, and let's get to the next point." The kids you deal with in tennis are usually well off and they're used to having their way, and when things don't go their way, they don't necessarily handle it well. We deal with kids whose families have spent $30 to $40,000 dollars a year on lessons. As I was coming here, I was talking to a very good friend of mine, and he was saying, let me know how it goes – he's got a daughter who is in tenth grade. So I think there is no doubt in my mind that for tennis purposes, what you're talking about is very important in how kids can let go of the negativity.*

I told Coach Minnis about my experience in my first sports hypnosis workshop, just as I described it to Coach Girouard in Chapter 7 regarding locking in good shots and flicking away bad ones, in order to focus only on the next play.

TM: *That's interesting. So how do you get them to focus? What are some of the methods you use?*

JT: *Well, I use hypnosis and teach them self-hypnosis to practice at home. It basically involves getting them to relax and concentrate and focus on whatever you, as coach, are telling them in training. And if there is negative self-talk, I need for them to tell me what that's all about and then I give them positive suggestions to counteract or reframe the negative. I tell the distance runner who is saying, "What was I thinking entering this distance race, I'm basically a sprinter?" to say, "Wait a minute, I'm a fine-tuned machine, I've been training for this, I'm in great shape. I'm a tough dude!"*

I also shared with the coach some of my experiences with other athletes such as golfers, including the one who had previously worked with Dr Rotella (see Chapter 2) and a volleyball player (see Chapter 9). I also mentioned to him the movie, *For Love of the Game*, and I was impressed that he was familiar enough with the movie that he quoted the verbal self-hypnotic instruction, "Clear the mechanism."

TM: *Tennis, more than any sport, involves negative self-talk. When I was competing myself, I'd fight the negative thoughts with "positive, positive, positive." And it's hard to explain this to the players. I tell them "push yourself mentally," which means to push the negative thoughts out and think positively. But it's a different time in terms of quick fix medicine, quick fix everything. It's hard to get them to focus on the journey and not just immediate results. I've coached for 19 years and find that the kids' lack of patience and lack of perseverance is worse than it was a few years ago. When things don't go their way, they have a really tough time handling it and they let it affect them emotionally. I find a difference in the "disconnect" too. I coached men in the past, and I find that guys can bounce back faster while with the girls, it just gets worse.*

JT: *I've been reading about Wimbledon and how a lot of the high seeds are losing to much lower seeds. Do you think a lot of that is mental?*

TM: *Well, Wimbledon is different – the surface is different. A lot of players are not good grass players – Venus is a great grass player. But the girl who just won the French Open – grass is not her forte.*

Coach Minnis went on to talk about the difference in venues, surfaces, and so on – for example, he explained how his LSU teams play well outdoors, but often compete successfully indoors. Likewise, Ohio State players play well indoors but they often struggle outdoors. He described how the really mentally tough players are those who can overcome these changes and play well regardless of the situation.

TM: *People don't understand why Pete Sampras or John McEnroe can't win on clay, or why Ivan Lendl can't win on grass. But it is all a mental thing. I think confidence in athletics comes from knowing in the back of your mind that you have done the right thing. And I think when you have character guys – your best players, from a team standpoint, who are working hard, practicing every day, staying out of trouble – those are the things that trickle down to the rest of the team. The character of knowing you have done the right things gives you more confidence in being successful. I've had a player or two with unbelievable talent as tennis players, but who are not of the best character and that trickles down in a negative way.*

I think in sports you need talent, but at some point in time you meet others with the same amount of talent, so what's going to make the difference? The difference is going to be your character, your work ethic, your ability to stay focused. I use the Saints with my team as an example, because they seem like a very solid, unselfish team. With some teams I've coached, we've done really well and it was a nightmare, and with others we've done okay, but it's been fun.

What people don't understand in sports, is whether you're number one in the country, or 10th or 30th, the ultimate is getting the most out of that team. So you might have a team that is 30th in the country that overachieves and does better than a team that was ranked 15th, because you got the most out of those players. That's what I see as character. And it's harder recruiting these days because of limits in contacts, so in a period of five or six days, I have to figure what I'm bringing in as far as character goes, and I think a lot of that is looking at the parents – you know, "The apple doesn't fall too far from the tree."

JT: *Tony, if I was working with one of your players, and I called you and said: "Coach, what things would you like me to reinforce hypnotically?", what would you want me to say?*

TM: *I think it is going to be a little different with each player. With some of them it would be the confidence to believe they can achieve. One of the things you have in tennis is a pecking order, so if I am rated higher in the country than you are, I believe that I can beat you. With other players it is the inner fighting that goes on and the consistency to focus over long periods of time. A lot of players are torn and can go from the highest high to the lowest low in a 10 minute span. They're fighting their emotions, and when you're doing that you can't focus on what you're trying to achieve. I'll give you a good example. When Roger Federer was coming up in the juniors, he was known for not having the tools, mentally, to be what he is capable of being, but somehow he gathered himself and matured and developed into one of the most mentally tough athletes, period, in any sport.*

JT: *Was it on Monday, at Wimbledon, when Federer was down two sets to none and he came back to pull out a win? After the first two sets, announcers on ESPN Sports Radio were saying one of the greatest upsets in the history of tennis was about to happen. Yet he came back. Was this just his mental toughness?*

TM: *Yes, I tell people this all the time: Federer has made 24 consecutive Grand Slam semi-finals. That's just unbelievable because you have a day like he had the other day – and that's over a six year time period, over all three surfaces. The amount of mental toughness it takes to achieve that is incredible. Because you're going to have off days, days when you're not feeling good, opponents whose style doesn't match well with yours, but to do that is unheard of. The next longest streak to his 24 is 10. He's amazing.*

In sports, having a short memory is so important in success or failure. Also imperative is trying to make these kids understand about this fear of failure, because their self-worth is so tied into success or failure. I try to get them to focus not so much on wins or losses, but on doing things consistently the right way. It is so important for players to be able to relax themselves after a bad shot and prepare themselves for the next one.

JT: *One of the chapters in my book is on recovering from injury and returning to competition. One day a week I work in a pain management* clinic. *I read about athletes who have the same injury, the same surgeon, and the same prognosis, but one returns to action and the other never plays again. Do you think this is all up here* (pointing to my head)?

TM: *Yes, I see that too. I had a girl playing for me who had been SEC champion the previous year, then got hurt and had arthritis develop in a facet in her back and couldn't play. I think part of it was she lost her desire, and part of it was that she was in pain. In her junior year she just wasn't very good, then in her senior year she played – but I think she was having some doubts about whether she wanted to play or not – and she played badly. Then she told me she was in the worst pain she had ever been in. So I benched her, and the next week she's telling me she feels so much better. We've been to the NCAA tournament for 14 of the last 15 years, but this year we didn't make it. And when the light came on that we were not going to make it, she came and asked to play. She won four matches at the end of the year and picked up her level of play and looked like her old self again. I tell my assistant all the time, from a psychological standpoint, so much is up here* (points to head). *Whether it be injury, whether it be attitude, negative self-talk is so much an important part of the psychology.*

Then I gave Coach Minnis a demonstration of the muscle testing technique.

TM: *That's amazing!*

The evening after that interview, at the top of the sports news was the story about how American John Isner, the 23rd seed, beat qualifier Nicholas Mahut, from France, in the longest ever tennis match at 11 hours and 5 minutes. It beat the previous longest match by almost five hours. After the winning shot, Isner reportedly dropped to his knees and Mahut hung his head for a moment. Isner obviously underplayed his true physical feelings as he told the Wimbledon crowd: "I got a little bit tired. Perhaps the adrenalin was still flowing." Mahut said: "At this moment, it is just really painful – but we played the greatest match ever." All I could think about was: "I wonder what Tony would have said about the mental toughness of these two guys?"

Case 1: The tennis player

Shortly thereafter, I was called by Tony Minnis' assistant coach. She said that a girl that Coach Minnis had talked with me about fell apart in a tournament in California, and she was now ready to start seeing me. Earlier in the year, this player, who was ranked 122st in the pre-season Intercollegiate Tennis Association (ITA) singles rankings, had beaten the 20th ranked player in three sets. Hopes were apparently very high for her in the California tournament, but things did not work out so well. She lost in her second singles match. In her first consult with me she described how she won the first set 6-2, but said: "In the second set I started freaking and my game broke down."

When posed the usual question about what percentage of her sport did she think was mental, she responded with 75 percent. She readily admitted that she spent little if any time, however, on mental training. The muscle testing technique described in previous chapters was employed with good results. We agreed to a schedule of four sessions over the next two weeks leading up to the next competition, which was the ITA Southern Regionals in Birmingham, Alabama.

First hypnotic session

I questioned the client further about that second singles match when she started "freaking out." She added: "I have a good serve and usually hold serve. But in the second match I didn't break her serve and then felt I had to hold serve and I didn't. I put a lot of pressure on myself." I asked what she did to try to regain composure, and she said: "I just tell myself to relax and have fun. It's just tennis, not life and death. I'm just really competitive – I really wanted to win and got mad at myself – not mad, but aggravated at how I was playing."

The first session was dedicated to getting her oriented to hypnosis with a primary focus on teaching her to relax. A reverse arm levitation technique was employed, followed by deep breathing exercises, then my usual first deepening approach using the elevator imagery. She was told about the practice effect and the generalization effect (also for ego strengthening), and I used three tests to ratify trance. The relaxation scenes were the beach scene, followed by the woods scene and the logjam image (described in Chapter 1). While she reported seeing nothing on the log, I conveyed to her that what was most important was her decision to take matters into her own hands to remedy the problem, to free up the blocks, so things could flow smoothly again. The interpretation was that this taking responsibility was symbolic of her coming to see me. She was then brought back to an alert state and given instructions regarding a three-step self-hypnotic approach to practice at home.

Second hypnotic session

At this meeting, the eye fixation induction was utilized, followed by deep breathing and the deepening technique involving descending a staircase. I then went directly into the World Class Visualizer technique (see Chapter 2). At first, when viewing her garden through the eyes and with the brain of a world class visualizer, she said nothing was really different. Then, however, she was able to describe the garden in much more detail and depth. When she described her tennis game, it was obvious that she knew what she needed to do in terms of being aggressive, staying focused, keeping her opponent on the defensive, pumping herself up, moving her feet, and playing with intensity. When she saw it through the eyes and with the brain of the world class expert in tennis, she saw it much the same, but making more first serves, playing more angles, and pumping herself up even more.

She later told me that she was emulating her coach from juniors who she saw as mentally tough. Before bringing her out of hypnosis, I talked with her about dealing with adversity and being able to put the past behind her and focus only on what is happening now.

Once out of hypnosis, we discussed techniques to lock in the good and flick off the bad. She indicated that she could lock in the good by slapping her leg, as she often did anyway, and get rid of the bad by tapping her racquet with her hand. She was also given the list of affirmations from the Appendix, and we decided we would make a CD at our next meeting.

Third hypnotic session

She was taught the eye roll induction followed by deep breathing and then a flexible deepening technique – allowing her to choose either an elevator ride, descending a staircase or escalator, or gently sloping hill – as I counted backwards from 10 to 1. The idea of approaching her sport with gratitude and thorough enjoyment was reinforced. She was told:

> I remember a number of years ago I was reading one of those in-flight magazines while traveling. There was an article about Larry Bird, who was then a great National Basketball Association star with the Boston Celtics. The interviewer commented that it must be a tough life having to be on the road so much during the season, being away from home, having to live in hotels, and so on. Larry responded: "Oh, yeah! I have to go to some great cities, stay in first class hotels, go out in the afternoon and shoot a few baskets, then at night go out and play my favorite game in the whole world, and get paid a lot of money for having fun. What a tough job!" So enjoy your opportunity to compete at a pretty high level in your sport.

As agreed, this session was recorded and a CD made for her.

Fourth hypnotic session

The client was given the choice to use whichever of the three previously introduced induction techniques she liked best. She chose eye fixation. This was followed by deep breathing exercises, and then the counting forwards technique of ascending an escalator up into the clouds (described in Chapter 2). The suggestion of looking down and seeing a time continuum was given. When looking into the past, she said she first started playing tennis at age 8 and it was fun. She was told to continue to approach her training and competition with the same enthusiasm.

When asked to focus on the more recent past, when she had played her most complete game, she talked about a few months earlier, in the team's first tournament of the year, when she beat the girl ranked 20th. She was told to concentrate on what she did right and learn from things that could have been done better. We talked about the idea of this being her baseline, or at least her potential, with suggestions that she could get even better. She was then asked: "Is it possible that you can play even better than that previous most complete game?" After she acknowledged that it was, I asked: "Well, if it is possible, then is it probable that you can play even better than that baseline performance?" She confirmed that it was.

Then, the Space Travel Meditation (described in Chapter 2) was used. She indicated that in her imagery she went to the moon, talked to the man on moon, and asked what she needed to do to play really well in the tournament that was coming up in three days time. She said the answer was: "Be focused and intense, but have fun and stay relaxed."

I followed the results on the internet and saw that she won against two different opponents on the Friday and one more on Saturday, thus making it to the quarter-finals. On Sunday she lost to the player ranked 20th whom she had beaten approximately two months earlier. Although this happened just before completing the writing of this book, and I have not had a chance to talk with my client, I was able to talk to her coach. He expressed disappointment. The fact that she had lost to someone she had beaten previously added to the frustration. He observed that it had nothing to do with her not being focused; rather, he said that it had to do with her not "playing smart." He observed that she sometimes plays "too big," instead of playing smart. This worked for her in the juniors, but at her present level it didn't and that playing smart was imperative. He said they had just got back from the tournament the night before and he had not yet had a chance to meet with her, but the match had been videotaped, and he intended to go over it with her when they met. My plan is not only to obtain this athlete's interpretation of what did not work, but to attempt to incorporate what Coach Minnis calls "playing smart" into the hypnotic suggestions.

Chapter 9

Volleyball, Soccer, Olympic Shooting, Cycling, and Rugby

Don't bother just to be better than your contemporaries or predecessors. Try to be better than yourself.

William Faulkner

These five sports are grouped together because I have had only limited experience in working with athletes in these areas. However, the results have been very positive. Volleyball, in particular, is a sport I often mention when talking about how the therapist need not have experience in the sport or even have worked with an athlete in that sport. As will be seen in the case example and in my interview of that player, who later coached at the collegiate level, my approach was to find out what concepts coaches attempt to convey to their players.

I worked with an Olympic shooting competitor and have had some experience with soccer, although I have never actually used hypnosis with a soccer player. In the US, rugby is not very popular, although I have one friend who played club rugby and some of the colleges in the Louisiana area have club teams. However, the ideas espoused throughout this book regarding not needing to know the sport in detail also hold true with these internationally popular sports. The idea is that the therapist needs only to interview the player and preferably his or her coach. The goal of the interview is to find out what suggestions can be presented hypnotically in the form of post-hypnotic suggestions that are consistent with what the coach is trying to instill.

Case 1: *The volleyball player*

Paige Huber-Pitts was referred to me by the mother of the high jumper/cheerleader referenced in Chapters 3 and 4. At the time, she was Paige Huber, a varsity volleyball player for the University of New Orleans (UNO). Now she is the mother of two boys aged 5 and 2 and about to deliver a third boy. Some of her accomplishments were unknown to me until I recently had the opportunity to interview her. Paige lettered at UNO for four years from 1997–2000. In the last three of those years she was selected to the Sun Belt Conference Academic Honor Roll.

Although a starter, she had not been playing up to expectations. I worked with her for three hypnotic sessions in the summer and fall of 1999, her junior year. The same methods and techniques described in earlier chapters with different sports were employed. In the week after our second session there was a write-up in the local newspaper in which she was prominently mentioned. The reporter noted that she'd had a career high in "digs," which I learned from her is a defensive maneuver that involves sacrificing your body by diving for the ball (this was on hardwood, not sand), and making a save before it touches the ground.

After one more session, I was invited to attend the team's next home game. What impressed me was that I watched this athlete practicing what she had learned. After a good play, she would lock it in by using the hand-tightening technique. If she felt she had made a mistake, she would get rid of it using the flick of the wrist and fingers. These signals were very subtle, as I had recommended, and perhaps no one else would have even noticed them. She reported that her ability to focus, and thus her total game, had greatly improved through the use of hypnotic techniques.

When I found out more about what Paige had been doing since I last saw her, I was especially interested in interviewing her. She had been an Assistant Volleyball Coach at UNO from 2002–2007, and is now the Athletic Director at Chapelle High School, where she had played on the team that won the Louisiana State Championship in 1995. So I was really keen to hear how she felt about the mental side of her sport and how the hypnotic experience helped her.

JT: *I would like to know how much you think our hypnotic training helped you, specifically, and in general your views about the mental side of volleyball.*

PHP: *As an athlete, I always was an anxious, nervous player. I started playing volleyball at 11, and this was the one and only sport I continued with all the way through. By the time I got to college, when we worked together, I was probably 20 or 21. I knew the mechanics because I had played so long. I was a defensive specialist. My role was digging and serve receiving. When you and I worked together we worked primarily on visualization, building confidence, and being able to focus and prepare for big moments in the game when I would be called on to perform my roles to the best of my abilities. The abilities were there; it was just learning to focus and do it perfectly. We worked on having the confidence to perfect the skills and to help my team.*

JT: *I remember watching you use the techniques of locking in the good plays and discarding the bad ones. And I remember you had a good game. I also remember being invited by the coach before the game to do a brief hypnotic induction with the whole team, but you guys lost. I assume that it was just a superior team and that the mental aspect is not what did it that day.*

PHP: *That year, 1999, was a transition year for us. We had a new coach and did not do very well. But the following year we played for the Sun Belt Conference Championship.* (The team's won-lost record in 1999 was 10-22, and only 5-11 in the Sun Belt Conference.)

JT: *Anything else you would like to add about the mental side of the game?*

PHP: *I remember that by doing the work with you it brought the physical side and the mental side together for me. You know, most athletes just work on the physical side of their game. Coaching staff will work on the mental part of team-building and bonding that will help get their athletes through the crucial parts, but they work very little on confidence and focus. I think volleyball is a very mental game. What can the hitter do to outsmart the other team's defense? How can the defender be ready for the opposing hitter's shot?*

When I coached in college and recruited, I looked at potential student athletes who were smart players – hitters who would know the correct shots to hit, setters who would know the correct hitter to set; an athlete who was an all-round student of the game as well as physically gifted enough to play at the collegiate level.

JT: *Well that makes sense since you were on the conference academic honor roll when you played, but I guess you are not talking about just book smarts?*

PHP: *Right, not just book smarts but understanding strategies of the game and being able to quickly put them into play. Some players can't — they just go into sensory overload. But the really good ones can.*

As mentioned earlier, although having had limited experience in working with volleyball players, this case example demonstrates how hypnosis and self-hypnosis can improve performance from the perspective of one player, who later went on to become an Assistant Coach at the college level and is now a high school Athletic Director. Volleyball seems to be a sport in which very little is written about the importance of mental focus. When I mentioned to Paige that I had found no literature on the subject with volleyball players, she indicated that she did not know of any either.

Case 2: The olympic shooter

I worked with a client a number of years ago who was an Olympic-class marksman. In our first session, he brought me a book to read about his sport. From this, I understood that marksmanship requires tremendous ability to block out distractions and to focus. I lost that book and his records in Hurricane Katrina, but as I remember it, after he came in for two sessions or so, he reported improvement in his ability to concentrate. He left the area to compete shortly thereafter, and I did not hear from him again.

I recall that although I did not know why, at the time this client reminded me of another I had seen around the same time. She was not an athlete, but expressed a great desire to learn to concentrate more deeply. I often tell this story to athletes when describing the power of concentration and focus:

I saw a woman who made her living as a telephone psychic. She told me that she did her readings with cards (not tarot cards, but regular playing cards), and she felt that by learning self-hypnotic techniques she would be better able to focus, block out distractions, and do more effective readings. She reported success after just a few sessions. Although her friend paid me for the hypnotherapy sessions, after the first one, she offered to give me a reading. She gave me predictions about things that would happen to me in the near future in each direction: north, east, south, and west. None of them came true. A few years later, however, I was contacted by an attorney friend who was having marital difficulties. She said she had talked with this psychic, and everything she predicted had come true. She brought over a tape of the session for me to hear how accurate the "reading" was. My internal response was: "Wow. She really has improved. Maybe the self-hypnotic training really did help her focus and concentrate." I remember talking to her just before the Miami Dolphins-Washington Redskins played in Super Bowl XVII in 1983. I asked her if she had any thoughts about who was going to win. She said that as a matter of fact, she had been having dreams of dolphins exhilaratingly jumping out of the water, making her think they would win. I said something to the effect of "Shucks, I was planning to make a friendly wager on the Redskins." To which she responded: "Well Joe, you know a lot more about football than I do, so why don't you go with your own intuition," which I did. I was happy to watch the Redskins win that game 27-17 after being behind 17-10 at halftime.

The message to be gleaned from this script is that we often know much more than we realize that we know – so be confident and "use what you know."

Soccer

I played soccer in my youth, around the age of 12 to 14 for a team in a YMCA city league. In those days, soccer was not a very popular sport in the US, nowhere close to how it is now. I was apparently pretty good at it because I made the winning goal in the City All-Star game. More recently, I became somewhat involved in my stepson's high school soccer playing. He was 15 when I met him and had been playing soccer since he was 4 years old. While

I never hypnotized him and did not want to get too directive in a sport in which he was much more accomplished than I, there were some talks about attitude that seemed to result in improved play and more starts. His team made it to the State Championship game in his senior year.

If I was asked to work with a soccer player, my approach would be very similar as with other athletes. That is, a first session to introduce the player to hypnosis and create a sense of optimism (muscle testing, test of visual imagery, trance ratification), and then to work on improved ability to relax and calm himself/herself. I would seek consultation with the player's coach regarding what areas needed a more focused, concentrated effort, and then I would reinforce these behaviors hypnotically. Visualizing the game with a positive outcome, and perhaps the Miracle Method would be effective. The Miracle Method is an approach which I first saw described by Miller and Berg (1995) in their book about using this technique with alcohol and drug addicts. It basically works as follows:

> I want you to imagine that you go to sleep tonight, as usual, but when you wake up in the morning, you realize that a miracle has occurred. Now, everything is just the way you have wanted it to be … Just as you have dreamed for it to be … Playing at your maximum potential … Take a little time to review what it is like … And especially how it is different than the way it used to be.

I typically wait two or three minutes, then say:

> So now tell me. What is different? How is it different? … So what happened that resulted in this miracle? … What changes had to occur in order for you to achieve this outcome?

This approach often enables the athlete to get a better perspective of their negative physical or mental approaches that need changing to foster more positive outcomes.

Cycling

While I have never worked with an elite cyclist, while talking about the upcoming publication of this book with a colleague, David Wark, he told me about a personal experience he had with biking. He is past-president of the American Society for Clinical Hypnosis (ASCH). While working with athletes is not really his thing, he wrote an article in the ASCH newsletter (Wark, 2008) about the First World Congress on Excellence in Sports and Life held in Beijing.

David used to have a bike and would ride 15–20 miles on a weekend, but his bike was stolen, so he got a slightly different type of bike, but it "just didn't move very fast." He added that one day a guy who did not appear to be very physically fit – he referred to him as "fat" – barreled past him on a plain looking bike. He said that he then began to "crank it up" until he passed him. It did something to his "whole biking system" and ever since then the bike just started going faster for him. He now realizes that there was obviously some negative self-talk going on about the change in bikes. This story was very similar to some of the personal vignettes I included in Chapter 3 regarding my experiences in distance running.

Since there are plans for me to begin working with a client who is a cyclist, I intend to use this story in addition to employing all of the methods described for use with other athletes.

Rugby

In the introduction, I made reference to the Association of Applied Sports Psychology (AASP) Annual Conference I recently attended. I was particularly interested in one presentation (Woodcock, et al., 2010) regarding their work with an elite youth rugby team in Scotland. One of the presenters was a coach from the Scottish Rugby Union. He described mental skills training as "the tools to cope" (i.e., relevant skills and methods that will enable players to survive and perform consistently under pressure and thrive on the national – and potentially international – stage in the future). Their research shows that the youth athletes not only reported improved performance in rugby, but were able to transfer the skills to other sports as well as to their life outside of sports (e.g., school).

In sum, all of the techniques, scripts, and stories used in this book can be applied to all sports including soccer, shooting, cycling, or rugby – indeed, any event that requires concentration, focus, and mental fine-tuning.

Chapter 10

Recovering from Injury and Returning to Training and Competition

If you think you are beaten, you are;
If you think you dare not, you don't.
If you'd like to win, but think you can't,
It's almost a cinch you won't.

If you think you'll lose, you're lost,
For out in the world we find
Success begins with a fellow's will;
It's all in the state of mind.

If you think you're outclassed, you are;
You've got to think high to rise.
You've got to be sure of yourself before
You can ever win a prize.

Life's battles don't always go
To the stronger or faster man;
But sooner or later the man who wins
Is the one who thinks he can.

(Attributed to Walter D. Wintle, a 19th century poet. The poem was originally titled "Thinking," but in later reprints was changed to "The Man Who Thinks He Can")

My work with pain patients (I currently work one day per week in a pain management clinic and am referred to as their "pain psychologist") dovetails nicely with working with athletes who have overuse or injury-related pain. For those sports psychologists not experienced with working with pain patients, they might familiarize themselves in this area by joining organizations that foster interdisciplinary pain treatment (for example, I belong to the Southern Pain Society and the Mississippi Pain Society). These organizations stress the importance of an interdisciplinary approach including orthopedics, pain management specialists (MDs, many of whom were originally trained in anesthesiology), psychologists, and physical therapists, among others.

A good starting place for review in this area is *Comprehensive sports injury management* by Jim Taylor et al. (2003) which addresses the psychological implications of injury, rehabilitation, and return to sport. Jim Taylor has been a consultant to the US and Japanese ski teams and is a former US top-20 ranked alpine ski racer who competed internationally. He is also a certified tennis-teaching professional and second degree black belt and certified karate instructor, a marathon runner, and an Ironman triathlete. He describes the importance of trust by the athlete in the sports medicine provider (pp. 27–28); as a result, I spend considerable time in the first meeting establishing rapport with my sports clients. This approach includes letting the athlete know that I am sensitive to their concerns and issues and I am there to help them attain their goals, not mine.

In a previous book, *Psychological approaches to sports injury rehabilitation* (1997), Jim and Shel Taylor point out how emotional factors such as loss of confidence and/or motivation and fear can be often harder to overcome than the physical injury itself.

Particularly beneficial for psychologists who use sports hypnosis with athletes is to have experience in reducing subjective pain with hypnosis. There are a number of hypnotic scripts that are effective for pain reduction in Hammond (1990), including some pre-surgery suggestions in Barber (p. 98) and Sylvester (pp. 98–101). There are also articles and books on the use of hypnosis to accelerate post-surgical healing (Hilgard and Hilgard, 1994; Eimer, 2002; Ginandes et al., 2003; Phillips, 2007) and related works on the mind–body connection as it relates to physical pain and healing (e.g., Rossi and Cheek, 1988). This combined approach allows the therapist to incorporate the two goals of pain reduction and improved performance in their work.

Just as with any client I see for pain management, I believe it is important to let the athlete with pain know that seeing a psychologist does not indicate that anyone thinks the pain is all in his or her head. The athlete in pain is told:

Of course if you did not have a brain, the pain would have nowhere to register, so in a way it is in your head, but no one doubts that you have a real injury that is causing the pain. After all, we have tests such as X-rays and MRI scans to show the area affected. But the psychology of pain may account for why some athletes adapt to the injury and pain and follow a normal course of recovery and others take longer.

I then tell clients two personal stories. The first involves my first American Society of Clinical Hypnosis (ASCH) workshop in St. Louis in 1978:

I was just learning to do hypnosis during an introductory workshop in 1978. One of the lecturers was teaching the entire group to do self-hypnosis. After the main lecture, we broke down into small discussion groups. I asked the instructor: "In the large group I was able to put myself into a trance state and imagine that the lower right quadrant of my back was a block of ice, numb and insensitive to pain. It worked in getting rid of the pain from a recent back injury. But as soon as I come out of trance the pain returns. How do you give yourself a post-hypnotic suggestion to remain pain free?" Her answer had nothing to do with hypnosis or self-hypnosis. She responded: "Well Joe, why do you need that pain?" I then realized that throughout the meetings, if I was very interested in what a particular speaker was saying, I was unaware of the pain. But when I became bored I felt the need to move to adjust my back and the pain was there. In her small group, there was one guy who I didn't like very much because he would try to dominate the discussion. Whenever he was speaking, I felt: "Damn, my back is hurting!" When the instructor spoke (who I liked), however, no pain! Now the injury was there and it showed up on X-rays, but how much I attended to it determined how much subjective pain I experienced.

The second story goes as follows:

After I became competitive in my age group in the 5k and 10k races put on by my local running club, I had a non-running related back injury. I had been cross-training with weights and was doing some arm exercises with relatively light dumbbells. When I went to put one of them down, reaching forward in an awkward position, I felt a pull in my back. By the next day the pain was pretty severe, so I went to see my chiropractor buddy who was an ultra-marathoner and who I had earlier helped quit smoking as it interfered with his effective running. He did some X-rays, diagnosing the condition as a vertebra out of place, and did chiropractic adjustments. He then told me to rest for a few days without any vigorous exercise. I said: "But I'm entered in a 5k race this Saturday (two days away) and I want to win." He asked: "Joe, could you just go out and run at a leisurely pace and not try to push yourself to compete?" I must have glared at him for a moment because he then said: "No, I guess you can't do that, can you? So just take four Ibuprofen before the race and go blow it out!" I followed his instructions, did well in the race, and felt no pain. Now I know that my injury and pain was not nearly as significant as what you are dealing with right now, but I think it is a good example of the power of the mind to compete if the motivation is strong enough. I don't want you to go against your doctor's or trainer's orders, I just want to help you to not fear competing within the boundaries they create for you.

In addition to the psychological aspects that determine the rapidity of return to sport, if the above-mentioned adaptation does not occur as fast as the prognosis has indicates it should, psychological symptoms such as anxiety, depression, and anger might develop. While relatively minor injuries may cause some emotional symptoms – because these are unexpected and seem uncontrollable – more serious ones often result in unfamiliar feelings and questions about whether the athlete will ever play again, or at least whether they will ever play so well.

I attempt to lessen subjective pain in much the same manner as with non-athletic pain. There are many scripts in Hammond (1990), but one that I often use is a modification of his Master Control Room technique which I have adapted for lowering subjective pain. The technique is just the same as described in Chapters 2 and 5, except with the golfer and equestrian athletes referred to in those chapters, the focus was on lowering anxiety. With pain patients, the monitor on the left is for pain, not anxiety. An exception is when the pain patient is also suffering from anxiety about their condition. In such cases, I have the client imagine two monitors on the left, side by side, one for pain and one for anxiety. Then, the process begins regarding turning up the relaxation control while lowering the control(s) on the left, decreasing pain or pain and anxiety, depending on the case.

Cellular healing script

For clients with injuries and anticipated surgery, I often use the following script (modified from Look, 1997) which I used in a case study for successful blepharoplasty using hypnosis and a local anesthetic (Tramontana, 2008b). It is useful for preparing clients for surgery and for recovery after surgery or injury.

As an athlete you have likely heard of muscle memory. This would mean that muscles have intelligence. Well, every cell in your body has intelligence. And that intelligence is what allows your body to heal. Think about it … Have you ever before broken a bone? *(If yes, continue. If not)* or known someone who has broken a bone? The patient usually goes to an emergency room or clinic. After X-rays and the resetting of the bone, it is likely put in a cast to immobilize that area. Then the patient is sent home for healing to begin. They are scheduled for periodic returns to the medical provider to check on progress, perhaps placement in a smaller cast, and so on, until they are discharged from medical care. Perhaps there is referral to a physical therapist. But it is not the doctor or cast technician or follow-up visits or physical therapist that does the healing. It is your body that heals itself, step by step, cell by cell. The body knows what to do and how to do it! The experiences with doctors, casts, and others only set the stage for healing to occur. But it is your body that heals itself, cell by cell, step by step.

Now, let's use another example: Let's say you or someone you know had a bad cut or laceration that needs stitches. You, or the patient if not you, likely goes to a hospital or clinic. A nurse cleans the wound. The doctor checks it out, then the doctor or nurse stitches the wound, perhaps puts ointment on it, then bandages it. The patient is then sent home with instructions for caring for the wound. But it is not the doctor or nurse or stitches or ointment or bandage that heals the wound. These things just set the stage for healing to begin. It is the patient's body that heals itself, step by step, cell by cell. So remember, your body knows what to do and how to do it.

Lingering injuries

It has long been a puzzle as to why some athletes with comparable conditions heal differently or at different rates. For example, two National Football League running backs who have the same knee injury (according to the diagnosis), the same surgeon, and the same prognosis for return to playing, but one returns to the game in the expected time or even sooner, and the other never plays again. Experts often theorize that the differences are mental. Taylor et. al. (2003) describe negative reactions by an athlete to an injury as normal to some degree because the condition or state is unfamiliar. If the player does not go through the regular adaptation processes and the injury lingers for longer than objective data indicates it should, a clinical condition likely has arisen. `

I had the good fortune to attend a workshop presented by Dr Dabney Ewin sponsored by the New Orleans Society for Clinical Hypnosis entitled "Ideomotor signals for rapid hypnoanalysis" (2008). At the time that I signed up for this seminar, I assumed that learning more about his approach would be of benefit to me in working with psychosomatic illness, especially psychosomatic pain management. I came to realize, however, that I could also adapt these techniques to my work with athletes with lingering injuries. In summary, Ewin teaches his patients ideomotor signals: that is, raising the index finger signals "yes," the long (middle) finger signals "no," and the thumb signals "I'm not ready to deal with that" or "I don't want to answer yet." At the workshop, and in his book of a similar title (Ewin and Eimer, 2006), he described "seven common causes" of psychosomatic disorders. These include conflict, organ language, motivation, past experience, identification, self-punishment, and suggestion. The theory is that since the left brain controls verbal behavior, logical and analytical thinking, and so forth, when questioned while in a hypnotic state, the client may still try to analyze what might be the most logical answer. The right brain, on the other hand, controls non-verbal behavior, creativity, reflexive or instinctive responding, and, in general, emotions or feelings. So his questioning always involves the phrases "do you feel" or "do you sense" that you are being affected by X? (for example, conflict). Kroger and Fezler (1976, p. 46) postulate that one cannot talk to the unconscious. Rather, they believe that Cheek's ideomotor signaling technique acts like a projective procedure and, as such, can elicit valuable information.

I had learned about ideomotor signaling many years ago and used it at times, but not in hypnotic uncovering of the origins of psychogenic disorders. One difference from Ewin's approach is that I always give an "I don't know" signal (the "pinky" finger). I ask that the client only use this as a last resort, since this response may make it too easy for them to avoid a "yes" or "no" signal. One observation that has always amused me is that when instructed to answer with their fingers, some clients would give a "yes" signal while nodding from side to side (a "no" response) or a "no" signal while nodding up and down.

After teaching the ideomotor signaling technique (Ewin and Eimer, 2006; Ewin, 2008), I say:

> One of the things that causes symptoms is what we call conflict. A conflict occurs when a person wants to do one thing and feels he or she should do the opposite. It is as if you feel you are being pulled in two directions. Answer with your fingers. Do you feel or sense that your problem in taking longer to heal and return to competition than the doctors expected is caused by conflict? *If he or she raises the yes finger, I ask:* Would it be alright for you to tell me about it? *If yes finger goes up, then:* Okay, tell me in your own words what you feel this conflict might be about.
>
> *Whether the answer was "yes" or "no," after reviewing the conflict, I go on:* Organ language is another thing that can cause symptoms. Organ language refers to phrases in our everyday conversation that include negative mention of a body organ like "I feel like I have been stabbed in the back," or "I feel like I am falling apart." Do you feel that organ language may be causing the symptoms? *If yes,* would it be alright to talk about it?
>
> *Next:* Another thing that may cause symptoms is motivation. A person can be motivated to have a symptom because it seems to solve some other problem; for example, a student who gets sick

at exam time or a soldier who does so before an impending battle. Now I know how badly you want to return to practice and competition, but do you feel or sense that in some way you may have a motivation to keep the pain? *(This can be very telling.)*

Next: Another possible cause of symptoms is past experience. An emotionally charged event may cause immediate onset of symptoms or sensitize you so that some other analogous event will activate the symptom. Do you sense or feel that your lingering injury problem started with a significant experience in your past? *If client responds affirmatively:* Would it be alright to go back and make a subconscious review of everything that was significant to you in this episode? *If he or she raises yes finger, I ask (depending on the current age of the client it might be necessary to begin at a lower age):* Did it happen before age 20? *If they indicate that it had not happened before age 20, I move forwards in five-year increments. If before age 20, I move backwards in five-year increments. Depending on the delineation of when it happened, I ask:* Is it alright to orient your mind to what happened before age X that relates to the present problem with difficulty getting over this injury?

Next: Another possible cause of symptoms is what we call identification. Do you feel that you are identifying with someone who had the same or similar symptom? *If the client gives an affirmative signal the usual line of questioning ensues.*

Then: Another possible cause of symptoms is self-punishment. Do you feel or sense that in some way your difficulty in healing and returning to competition is a form of self-punishment? *And again, questioning follows using finger signals until the client is asked:* Would it be alright to talk to me about this issue?

And finally: Yet another cause for continuing the symptom is suggestion. For example, do you sense or feel that someone in your past may have given you a negative suggestion that is affecting your return to practice and competition? *If yes:* Would it be alright to bring this up to a conscious level and discuss this suggestion? *If no, I do some prodding, because I often see this factor as a cause for self-doubt and even self-sabotage.* For example, if someone in your past ever suggested that you would never be successful, or would never amount to anything … Could this be the case?

In summary, ideomotor signaling can help the therapist gain some insights about the psychodynamic causes of the client's problems and assist in formulating a treatment plan. Once again, I recommend a somewhat eclectic approach that includes hypnosis for "uncovering" (i.e., age regression) and/or hypnoanalysis via ideomotor signaling, cognitive-behavioral techniques, reframing and other neurolinguistic programming approaches, guided imagery, and any other techniques in the therapist's repertoire that will enhance return to sport after an injury.

Chapter 11

Substance Abuse and Other Addictive Behaviors

A bend in the road is not the end of the road,
unless you fail to make the turn.

Anonymous

I suggested in Chapter 10 that some experience with pain management is helpful in working with athletes who are injured. I also believe that some knowledge of addictions is useful when working with athletes who develop maladaptive patterns such as drug and alcohol use and abuse. Therapists using sports hypnosis need not be an expert in addictions, but should have a firm base in how to treat or make appropriate referrals for these conditions. See also my book on hypnotically enhanced treatment of addictions (Tramontana, 2009a).

In 1983, I was invited to be a guest on the Wayne Mack radio show. Mr Mack was a long-time, very highly regarded talk radio host on a New Orleans station. In this particular show, his topic was cocaine abuse in professional sports. I must admit that in those days I was not very well versed in this area, although I had considerable experience in working with non-athlete drug abuse, so some research was in order. I could not find much literature on this topic at the time, but a helpful book was published a few years later by Gary Wadler and Brian Hainline called *Drugs and the athlete* (1989).

One of the most commonly discussed issues in the media at present is performance-enhancing drugs (usually anabolic steroids). It is unclear if this represents a true addiction or simply an obsession with getting better, stronger, faster, and so on – as well as ignorance of (or disregard for) the negative health consequences or the penalties for getting caught.

A number of famous athletes appear to be neither ignorant nor uncaring about sanctions and penalties but have got caught anyway. These include the track star Marion Jones and the cyclist Lance Armstrong. A number of famous football players, especially professional offensive linemen, and baseball stars – such as Mark McGuire, who allegedly set the home run record while using performance-enhancement drugs, Barry Bonds, Alex Rodriguez (A-Rod), and Manny Ramirez – have also been in the spotlight.

Athletes abuse steroids because they improve strength and performance. Rational scientific explorations into the mechanism of this effect and possible medical complications are limited because abusers routinely take doses that far exceed what any doctor would ethically administer. In the early 1990s, competitive athletes stopped using Nandrolone, although it was considered effective, because it remained in the body for weeks and was therefore very responsive to testing. Precursors of Nandrolone, such as 19-Norandrostenenedione and 19-Norandrostenediol, which were sold legally in health food stores, became the substitute for Nandrolone. However, they are rapidly converted to Nandrolone and still would lead to disbarment if an athlete tested positive (Karch, 2009, pp. 611–612).

In the past, various types of speed (amphetamines) were used to stimulate performance. Painkillers have been known to cause addiction in some famous players. For example, the All-Pro, Super Bowl winning quarterback, Brett Farve, admitted having become addicted to painkillers that allowed him to play each week (King, 1996). He completed a rehabilitation program and that facility now has a new gym, which I am told he paid for as a donation to the program.

In 2009, the great Olympic swimming star of the 2008 Summer Olympics, Michael Phelps, made the news after being caught on film smoking marijuana. He was suspended from competition for a spell. On one day in May, 2009, the local sports page had three references to athletes who were in trouble because of drugs or alcohol. There was a story about NASCAR driver Jeremy Mayfield being suspended for testing positive for an unnamed drug; a brief note about Donte Stallworth, wide receiver for the Cleveland Browns and formerly a very high draft choice of the New Orleans Saints, who was free on bail on a driving-under-the-influence manslaughter charge from March 2009 when he struck and killed a man; and a report about National Football League receiver Reggie Williams, who had pled guilty and was given two years probation for cocaine possession in a case in which a Taser was used to subdue him. Stallworth faces a 15-year prison sentence if he is convicted.

Then there are the illicit drugs. The basketball player, Len Bias was predicted to be a fantastic pro, but died from a cocaine overdose in 1986 after being drafted and before ever playing a professional game. Wadler and Hainline (1989, pp. 4–11) list many athletes who have died from drug overdoses, and many more whose careers were shortened because of drug abuse. They observed that the cocaine-related deaths in 1986 of Len Bias and Don Rogers, a football player with the Cleveland Browns, were a major impetus to drug-testing in sports. During the 1980s, cocaine was the number one drug abused, but unlike amphetamines it was used more for social reasons than for performance enhancement.

Karch (2009) describes the ergogenic effects of caffeine. Studies show that it improves performance and endurance during prolonged, exhaustive exercise such as cycling or long-distance running. He notes that sports governing bodies, such as the International Olympics Committee, ban excessive use of caffeine; however, even without exceeding their 12 mg/ml limit, performance improvement has been demonstrated with marathon runners. In short-term competition, with intense aerobic exercise of greater than 90 percent VO_2 max (maximal oxygen consumption), improved time to exhaustion has been repeatedly confirmed, although the performance increment has not been so great. In the 1990s, a great deal was written about the dangers of combining caffeine with ephedra/ephedrine in athletic supplements, and the increased risk of such combinations for producing cardiovascular disease (Karch, 2009, p. 222).

Tobacco addiction

While cigarette smoking is now uncommon in athletes, it does still occur. I have worked at different times with two marathon runners who were still smoking cigarettes and came to see me for smoking cessation hypnosis (see Tramontana, 2009a). While common wisdom says that when runners begin endurance training they often decide to quit smoking on their own, these two individuals were still smoking. Neither were elite runners, but the female had run a few and the male had run several marathons. After quitting smoking, the male runner went on to run many more marathons and even some ultra-marathons.

The male marathoner, a local health-care provider, was approached by a journalist from the local newspaper. It was National Smoke-Out Day, and she was preparing a story. She said that she knew that he was a marathon runner who used to smoke and wondered if he could help her readers by letting them know how he quit. He told her: "You need to go interview Dr Joe Tramontana. He is the one who taught me to quit through hypnosis." The reporter did follow up with me and wrote a really nice piece. I got more referrals from that article than any I ever paid for.

Eating disorders

Jockeys are infamous for having eating disorders. To maintain a low enough weight level, they often use a variety of techniques to maintain their weight, including purging. In *Helping athletes with eating disorders*, Ron Thompson and Roberta Sherman (1993) observe:

> We are reminded that people often think athletes are healthier than the general population. It is ironic, then, that the same characteristics that contribute to their prowess, along with aspects of their training and exercise, may also contribute to the development of eating disorders in too many athletes.

They suggest that getting in shape is too often associated with restrictive dieting, and we need to somehow put real health back into the eating and exercise regimens of athletes.

In summary, individuals who want to improve sports performance but also have drug use and addiction problems can be treated using hypnotic techniques for both, although not necessarily in the same sessions. And just as when working with athletes with injury and pain, a psychologist working with a client for improved sports performance might only later realize they are using/abusing substances, but the transition to focus on that problem can be easy. Likewise, those athletes who are first referred or self-refer for drug issues can later be worked with to improve sports performance.

The quote at the beginning of this chapter regarding the bend in the road not being the end of the road unless you fail to make the turn reminds me of a story I tell many of my addict clients (Tramontana, 2009a):

> An author who wrote a book about recovery from addiction talked about how he had been working with a group of addicts. He said one of the guys in his group never spoke, not even a word. One day, while talking with the group about choices as it relates to their decisions about using drugs, he told them that it is just like driving a bus. When you get to an intersection and must stop, you can then decide either to turn right, turn left, go straight ahead, or even do a U-turn and go back the way you came. He said the quiet client finally broke his silence. It was as if a light bulb went off in his head, and he said: "I finally understand my problem. All of these years I've had a junkie driving my bus."

While this story is told with the intention of introducing some levity into sessions, when dealing with athletes, especially at the professional level, the cost of using can be millions of dollars – and, of course, wasting a career and potential, as well as the money, is not the least bit funny.

Conclusion

Do just once what others say you can't do and you
will never pay attention to their limitations again.

James R. Cook

As noted in the Introduction, there are many areas in which hypnotic techniques can aid in performance enhancement. In my clinical practice, I have frequently used it successfully with clients who have a fear of public speaking or stage fright. Recently, a depressed and anxious adolescent, who also happened to be a ballet dancer, asked if the techniques we used for decreasing anxiety could help her ballet performance. After one session focusing on seeing herself performing just as her instructor had been working with her to achieve, she reported that it helped greatly.

For a long time, I have worked with students – from adolescents to adults returning to school for continuing education – on hypnotic techniques to improve study habits and exam taking. Recently, I worked with a young man who had been an honors student but was having trouble getting a high enough ACT score to go to the college he wanted to attend. He had already taken the test several times, always scoring a couple of points shy of the entrance requirement for that university. It was obvious that he had the ability but was suffering from test-taking anxiety. After one hypnotic session, a few days before the next scheduled test, he scored above the required level for admission. He and his family attribute this success to his hypnotic experience.

My recent attendance of a presentation by Wark (2009) on alert, open-eyed hypnosis, has added to my repertoire in working with individuals whose performance situation is inconsistent with eyes closed. Although I intend to continue starting with traditional eyes-closed inductions, I plan to continue refining how I incorporate his techniques into transitioning the client from closed eye to open eye hypnosis.

There has been some recent discussion about healing without formal hypnotic suggestions. Gafner (2008) states: "People have resources within themselves to help solve their problem." A couple of recent clinical experiences reinforce this idea. I had an anesthesiologist come to see me for bruxism. He was not only grinding his teeth at night, but he was clenching and grinding throughout the day and said that his coworkers had often commented on it (apparently, it was quite annoying). The first meeting was spent on information gathering and with an orientation to hypnosis, and although time was running short I wanted to give him something to leave with that would offer him some optimism for the future. I said:

> Because of time limitations, today I am just going to focus on teaching you to relax. We won't have time today to get into specific hypnotic suggestions to decrease or eliminate jaw clenching and teeth grinding, but we will do that in our next session.

After teaching him the relaxation techniques described in Chapter 1 (the beach scene, the woods scene with the logjam imagery), he was taught self-hypnotic techniques and was scheduled to return the following week. At the next session, however, he announced: "I'm cured. Did you give me some imbedded suggestion to stop my grinding? Because it has stopped. People at work even noticed." My interpretation was as follows: "No, I did not. I just taught you how good you are at getting into a relaxed state. My theory is that your own unconscious mind knew what to do and how to do it. So hypnotic relaxation merely set the stage for you to heal yourself."

Shortly after that, I had a referral from a neurologist. When I saw the patient in the waiting room, I wondered if I would be able to help her. She had severe upper body spasms and jerking. I have worked with tics before but this seemed much more extreme than anything I had seen previously. Her sister was filling out her paperwork because she jerked too much to write. I learned afterwards that the referring neurologist had told my receptionist when making the appointment: "If Dr T. can fix this one, he is a miracle worker."

The first meeting was much like that with the bruxism patient above. I told her before beginning hypnosis that time limits would not allow us to get directly into suggestions regarding the body jerking, and we would do that in her next session. I said that this time we were just going to concentrate on pure relaxation. By the time we finished the deep breathing exercises, much of the jerking had stopped. When we finished the visual imagery of the relaxing scenes, it had ceased completely. I told her we would do more work next time we met. When we walked out to the reception desk to schedule her next appointment, my receptionist looked at the patient, realized the change, and exclaimed: "Oh my God, you are a miracle worker." The client sat in the waiting room for an additional 45 minutes waiting for her sister to return. According to the receptionist, she sat reading a book without even a hint of jerking. She returned the next week with a slight tic, but by the end of the session it had resolved.

The illustrations of the unconscious solving our clients' problems not only reinforces the message of the cellular healing script (Chapter 10) on returning from injury, but it applies to all athletes. For example, suggestions are given that the unconscious mind already knows what to do and how to do it. Their coaches have taught them well regarding the mechanics of their sport. Now they are learning to use what they know.

A recent experience may greatly improve my ability to work with athletes at all levels who are on road trips, away tournaments, or tours (which do not allow them to come in as regularly as might be ideal or to have contact during the off times of a competition). A weight-loss patient had come to see me in my Baton Rouge office and agreed to pay in advance for a 20-session package (in order to receive a cash discount on her total treatment costs). As noted in Tramontana (2009a), I typically have smokers pay up-front for a three-session package, for which they receive a 20 percent discount. With weight loss, the number of sessions depends on the amount of weight the client wants to lose. This particular client had been making progress, but after the tenth session informed me that she was moving to Houston. By then, we were on a once per month schedule. Her company's home office was in Baton Rouge, so she wished to plan her monthly sessions on a day when she was in town for business. After a couple of times doing it this way, then some cancelled appointments because of meetings, schedule changes, and the like, she asked if we could have telephone sessions. She also requested that we increase the frequency to weekly, because there had been some regression.

I informed her that I had never hypnotized anyone by telephone, but since we had worked together for a while and she was experienced with my techniques and style, I would be willing to give it a go. After the first such phone session, we both felt it went well and scheduled future sessions at the same time and on the same day of the week. This approach, according to the client's report of further and steady weight loss, appears much more effective than a tape of my voice, which would not allow for the flexibility of changing suggestions as the situation calls for modifications. While I would not advocate this approach for working with new clients, it might be a good option for those who have hypnosis experience with a therapist but for whom travel does not allow the ideal frequency or regularity of sessions. Since that experience, I have employed brief, long distance telephone consultations with both the young golfer (in Chapter 2) and the intercollegiate equestrian (in Chapter 5) with good success.

When I give talks about hypnotically enhanced treatment approaches whether with addictions (Tramontana, 2008a, 2009b, 2009c) or other clinical issues (Tramontana, 2005), I caution workshop participants: "Do not teach self-hypnosis to sociopaths!" I tell the story of a patient I saw quite some time ago who had been in considerable trouble with the law (let's just say the Feds were paying for his treatment). In fact, he was quite the con man. He was referred for anger outbursts such as pulling phone lines out of the wall, breaking furniture, and his wife was about to leave him. I thought that surely I would be able to improve the situation by teaching him self-hypnotic techniques to calm himself in situations that caused rage. He was a quick study, and his presenting problem quickly resolved. His wife, however, came with him for a session and said: "Dr T., my husband is doing much better with the anger, but you need to tell him that he can't go around hypnotizing the whole neighborhood."

Someone close to me called recently and gave me a reminder that perhaps another caution is in order. She had rung the day before asking if I could help her feel less anxious regarding an upcoming dance recital. She said that she knew I was writing a book on sports hypnosis and wondered if it might work with dancing. She had been in an adult jazz dance class for years, and she said that every year as the recital got closer she would begin to panic. I did not do formal, long distance hypnosis with her, but I thought I could help. I told her that when we got off the phone she should put herself into a relaxed meditational state and mentally rehearse the entire dance from start to finish – see herself doing it just as she would like to do it. I explained that in this way she was mentally rehearsing success instead of mentally rehearsing failure, as she had been doing, which led to the feelings of anxiety. When she called the next day, she said: "You had better include a caution in your book about people with obsessive-compulsive disorder. I practiced the mental rehearsal over and over and over, until 5 a.m. and today I am exhausted."

I had forgotten to give her the standard post-hypnotic suggestion that after you do the mental rehearsal to give yourself the suggestion that you are going to continue relaxing for a specified amount of time, after which you will open your eyes, wide awake, alert, refreshed, calm and confident. Furthermore, I realized that with clients who have obsessive-compulsive traits, some limits should be suggested regarding the amount of repetition and the time spent doing them. We tend to focus on recommending a certain number of times to practice self-hypnosis, without consideration that an obsessive-compulsive person might take this to an extreme. This response would be especially counter-productive the night before a competition or performance, resulting in physical fatigue and diminished performance.

A note on marketing

As I reported in earlier chapters, I have tried several marketing approaches in the past, with little success. These included letters to coaches, a presentation to the athletic department at the University of New Orleans, and a free seminar on sports hypnosis that was advertised in the local newspaper. The latter was done with the assistance of a good friend (and avid golfer) who also has an advertising agency. That seminar was attended by one high school athlete, who I was already seeing for behavioral issues, not for sports performance, and his father (a former athlete).

However, after deciding to interview some coaches in sports in which I had not previously worked with any athletes, I mailed letters to a number of coaches at Louisiana State University. Two of these coaches responded (women's tennis and softball). A third coach was contacted via a mutual acquaintance. In all of these cases, I explained that I was writing this book and would like to pick their brains about how they saw the mental side of their particular sport. Fortuitously, I learned that just by the fact that these coaches responded to this request, it indicated an interest in the mental side of their sport. One of the coaches even commented that she wished she had brought her own tape recorder so she would be able to remember everything we talked about. She definitely saw the interview as a learning experience for herself as well as for me.

All three of these coaches have indicated a desire to send one or more of their athletes to see me, and two of the case examples (one equestrian and one tennis player) referred to in earlier chapters were the results of these interviews. I expect that as the coaches see improvement in their athletes, more referrals will be forthcoming.

My experiences with these individuals suggests to me that coaches would be very helpful if asked for an interview regarding the mental side of their sport (with the implied message of a desire to work with athletes in that sport). The outcome might well be consistent with what I have experienced. Once the coach has a better understanding of the positive effects of hypnosis, they very well might want their own athletes to have this "mental edge." In this way, the interview with the coach serves to educate them about hypnosis while also learning from them about the mental aspects of their sport. So far, the results have been positive.

To conclude, I hope you have realized that what I said in the Introduction is obviously true. I find it delightful to work with athletes. They usually do not have serious psychopathology issues (except those addicted to or abusing drugs). They are typically energetic, motivated, and willing to practice self-hypnotic techniques and do whatever it takes to improve their performance, and changes are often measurable and dramatic.

Appendix

Affirmations

I give athletes the following list of motivational quotations and suggest they pick and choose what works for them as an affirmation. Some of the quotes are attributed to more than one person. For example, both Thomas Jefferson and Benjamin Franklin are attributed with: "I'm a strong believer in luck and I find the harder I work, the more of it I have." And several individuals are credited with the statement: "Luck ... When preparation meets opportunity." One saying that I find somewhat amusing is a quote from famous former National Football League coach, Don Shula, who said: "Sure, luck means a lot in football. Not having a good quarterback is bad luck!"

> Ability is what you are capable of doing. Motivation determines what you do. Attitude determines how well you do it.
>
> Lou Holtz

> A bend in the road is not the end of the road, unless you fail to make the turn.
>
> Anonymous

> Do just once what others say you can't do and you will never pay attention to their limitations again.
>
> James R. Cook

> Don't be afraid of failing because of a mistake; be afraid of failing to learn from a mistake.
>
> Anonymous

> Don't be discouraged by a failure. It can be a positive experience. Failure is, in a sense, the highway to success, inasmuch as every discovery of what is false leads us to seek earnestly after what is true, and every fresh experience points

out some form of error which we shall afterwards carefully avoid.

John Keats

Don't bother just to be better than your contemporaries or predecessors. Try to be better than yourself.

William Faulkner

Efforts and courage are not enough without purpose and direction.

John F. Kennedy

An error doesn't become a mistake until you refuse to correct it.

Orlando A. Batista

Excellence is the result of caring more than others think is wise, risking more than others think are safe, dreaming more than others think is practical and expecting more than others think is possible.

Anonymous

Great love and great achievements involve great risk.

Anonymous

Great minds have purposes, little minds have wishes.

Washington Irving

The greatest mistake you can make in life is to be continually feeling you will make one.

Albert Hubbard

The greatest pleasure in life is doing what people say you cannot do.

Walter Bagehot

He who is outside his door has the hardest part of his journey behind him.

Dutch proverb

The highest reward for a person's toil is not what she gets for it, but rather what she becomes by it.

Anonymous

I am not competitive. I simply win.

Colorado Jules

I don't know the key to success, but the key to failure is trying to please everybody.

Bill Cosby

I honestly think it better to be a failure at something you love than to be a success at something you hate.

George Burns

If one advances confidently in the directions of his dreams, and endeavors to live the life which he has imagined, he will meet with a success unexpected in common hours.

Henry David Thoreau

If we all did the things we are capable of, we would astound ourselves.

Thomas Edison

If you can't do extraordinary things, do ordinary things extraordinarily well.

Anonymous

If you can't win, make the fellow ahead of you break the record.

Anonymous

If you find a path with no obstacles, it probably doesn't lead anywhere.

Frank A. Clark

In the middle of a difficulty lies opportunity.

Albert Einstein

It had long since come to my attention that people of accomplishment rarely sat back and let things happen to them. They went out and happened to things.

Elinor Smith

It is better to begin in the evening than not at all.

English proverb

It is never too late to be what you might have been.

George Eliot

It is not a tragedy to have only one talent; the tragedy is in not using it.

Farmer's Almanac

It is not because things are difficult that we do not dare, it is because we do not dare that things are difficult.

Seneca

It's not who you are that holds you back, it's who you think you're not.

Anonymous

Keep away from people who try to belittle your ambitions. Small people always do that, but the really great make you feel that you, too, can become great.

Mark Twain

Life is 10 percent what happens to you, and 90 percent how you respond to it.

Anonymous

Listen to your heart and proceed with confidence.

Anonymous

A man must be big enough to admit his mistakes, smart enough to profit from them and strong enough to correct them.

John C. Maxwell

No one can predict to what heights you can soar. Even you will not know until you spread your wings.

> Anonymous

Nothing great was ever achieved without enthusiasm.

> Henry David Thoreau

Obstacles are those frightful things you see when you take your eyes off your goal.

> Henry Ford

One important key to success is self-confidence. An important key to self-confidence is preparation.

> Arthur Ashe

The only thing in life achieved without effort is failure.

> Anonymous

Only those who dare to fail greatly can ever achieve greatly.

> Robert F. Kennedy

Only those who do nothing make no mistakes.

> Anonymous

Opportunity dances with those who are already on the dance floor.

> H. Jackson Brown

Our doubts are traitors and make us lose the good we oft might win by fearing to attempt.

> William Shakespeare

The power of fortune is confessed only by the miserable, for the happy impute all their success to prudence or merit.

> Jonathan Swift

Practice makes perfect, so be careful what you practice.

> Anonymous

Progress is not created by contented people.

Frank Tyger

Put your heart, mind, intellect and soul even to your smallest acts. This is the secret of success.

Swami Sivananda Saraswati

A smooth sea never made a skillful sailor.

Anonymous

Success is a lousy teacher. It seduces smart people into thinking they can't lose.

Bill Gates

Success is measured not by what you gain, but what you overcome.

Anonymous

Success is not measured by what you accomplish. It's measured by the opposition you encounter, and the courage with which you maintain your struggle against the odds.

Jerry Frenz

Success is that old ABC – ability, breaks, and courage.

Charles Luckman

Take calculated risks. That is quite different from being rash.

General George S. Patton, Jr.

There are no mistakes, only lessons.

Anonymous

There are no secrets to success. It is the result of preparation, hard work, and learning from failure. The person who really wants to do something finds a way; the others find an excuse.

Colin Powell

Trouble is merely opportunity dressed in work clothes.

Anonymous

Victory is sweetest when you've known defeat.

Anonymous

The vision must be followed by the venture. It is not enough to stare up the steps – we must step up the stairs.

Vance Havner

We are what we repeatedly do. Excellence, then, is not an act, but a habit.

Aristotle

Whatever you do, or dream you can, begin it. Boldness has genius and power and magic in it.

Goethe

When I stand before God at the end of my life, I would hope that I would not have a single bit of talent left, and could say, "I used everything you gave me."

Erma Bombeck

When you lose, don't lose the lesson.

Anonymous

Whether you think you can or think you can't, you're right.

Henry Ford

You can do whatever you have to do, and sometimes you can do it even better than you think you can.

Anonymous

You can't build a reputation on what you're going to do.

Anonymous

You can't win if you don't begin.

Anonymous

You have succeeded in life when all you really want is only what you really need.

Vernon Howard

You must have long-range goals to keep you from being frustrated by short-range failures.

Charles C. Noble

You shouldn't compare yourself to the best others can do.

Anonymous

You'll always miss 100 percent of the shots you don't take.

Anonymous

You're never as good as everyone tells you when you win and you're never as bad as they say when you lose.

Lou Holtz

Recommended Books and Movies

The following books and movies are often recommended to athletes, depending on their individual situations. For ease of reference, except for one book listed as "General," they are presented in the order of the chapters with their respective sports, beginning with Chapter 2.

The movies, however, are all bunched at the end since most of them have inspirational values that generalize across all sports.

General

Mack, G. and Casstevens, D. (2001). *Mind gym: an athlete's guide to inner excellence*. Chicago, IL: Contemporary Books

> This was recommended by Coach Girouard as the single book she most recommends to athletes. The foreword is written by baseball great Alex Rodriguez. One of the pre-publication reviews was done by former Vice-President Dan Quayle, who is described as a 4-handicapper. He says: "As an avid golfer, I recommend this book to anyone desiring to raise their productivity or to lower their handicap." Jason Kidd, NBA All-Star and Olympic gold medalist with the US Basketball Team said: "I read *Mind Gym* on my way to the Sydney Olympics and really got a lot out of it. Gary has important lessons to teach, and you'll find the exercises fun and beneficial."

> Gary Mack is a noted sports psychologist who has worked with professional athletes in most major sports. He explains how your mind influences your athletic performance as much as does your physical skill, if not more so. The book includes 40 lessons and inspirational anecdotes from prominent athletes, many of whom he has worked with to build "mental muscle."

Chapter 2: Golf

Gallwey, W. T. (1981). *The inner game of golf*. New York: Random House

> Tim Gallwey has written three previous books on tennis and skiing and his "inner game concepts" have been accepted in many sports as well as other areas of life. The general thesis is that one's mind, emotions, and confidence play a much larger role in golf than in almost any other sport. It is noted that in tennis, the player is hitting and moving the ball over and over again while on the run, and in skiing the skier is hurdling down a mountain, so their reactions are much more instinctual than intellectual. He adds that in 18 holes of golf, the player actually hits the ball for no more than three or four minutes during a four-hour round, and it is the time between the shots that is the bane of the average player. Whether he is brooding over having flubbed his last drive, dreading his next shot from a sand trap, or trying to line up the tricky six-foot putt, he is constantly grappling with self-doubt, fear of failure, tension or even anxiety.

Rotella, R. (1995). *Golf is not a game of perfect*. New York: Simon & Schuster

> This is a book written for players. It is filled with delightful and insightful stories about golf and the golfers with whom Dr Rotella has worked. He was the Director of Sports Psychology for 20 years at the University of Virginia and now consults with many of the world's leading golfers as well as some of the top golf organizations including the PGA, LPGA, and Senior LGPA.

Rotella, R. (1996). *Golf is a game of confidence*. New York: Simon & Schuster

> This book is filled with anecdotes and inspirational instruction. It focuses on the most important skill a golfer can have, the ability to think confidently. Dr Rotella helps readers revolutionize their own mental game and approach to course management, and he relates stories of the game's legendary figures. In other words, he not only allows the reader to get inside the ropes, but also to get inside the heads of the game's greatest players in their most important moments.

Rotella, R. (2004). *The golfer's mind.* New York: Simon & Schuster

This book was actually first suggested to Dr Rotella by Davis Lowe, Jr., Davis Lowe, III's dad, who encouraged him to write an instructional book on golf's mental challenges, organized by topic. He thought that golfers should keep the book nearby at all times so that when they needed a refresher on a certain issue, they could consult the book, read it for a few minutes, and take away guidance regarding their difficulties. He gives his ten commandments of achieving peak performance which range from (1) Play to play great. Don't play not to play poorly, to (10) Love your wedge and your putter.

Saunders, T. (2005). *Golf: lower your score with mental training.* Carmarthen, UK: Crown House Publishing

Tom Saunders, MD focuses on overcoming bad habits/swings by training your mind. His approach involves focusing completely on the shot you are about to take, developing positive thoughts and behavior patterns, using mental imagery to improve your game, and achieving active relaxation. The book is also accompanied by a CD of exercises focused on creating peak performance in golf and in other sports.

Chapter 3: Running

Galloway, J. (2001). *Marathon: you can do it!* Bolinas, CA: Shelter Publications

The focus of this book is to prepare runners of all abilities to train safely and complete a marathon using his principles.

Galloway, J. (2002). *Galloway's book on running* (2nd edn). Bolinas, CA: Shelter Publications

In this excellent book, written by one of the editors and feature writers of *Runner's World Magazine,* Jeff Galloway – whose first book sold over 400,000 copies after being published in 1984 – is described as a world-class runner who decided in the 1980s that his mission in life was to teach others how to run and make fitness a permanent part of their lives. In this edition, besides training programs for preparing for a marathon, he adds training tips and strategies for 5K to half-marathon distances. He also places particular emphasis on the needs of the older runner, with an emphasis on fat burning and the importance of rest.

Higdon, H. (1997). *How to train: the best programs, workouts, and schedules for runners of all ages.* Emmanus, PA: Rodale Press

> Hal Higdon presents an excellent compendium of techniques and strategies for runners of all ability levels, as well as ages.

McDougall, C. (2010). *Born to run: a hidden tribe, superathletes, and the greatest race the world has never seen.* New York: Knopf

> Jeff Galloway, the author of the books referenced above, wrote a review for this which says: "Having been a runner for over fifty years, I appreciate and enjoy the characters in Christopher McDougall's *Born to run.* These are real people who express their addiction to running in quirky ways." It is a very inspirational book about how the author found the Tarahumara Indians of Mexico's Copper Canyons who run hundreds of miles without rest and chase down anything from a deer to an Olympic marathoner while enjoying every minute of it. Reading the book will make you want to run (or, in my case, to start running again).

Sandrock, M. (2001). *Running tough.* Champaign, IL: Human Kinetics

> In the preface, Michael Sandrock refers to a training run at high altitude involving Steve Prefontaine and Frank Shorter, both world-class runners. Prefontaine was already a world-champion at three miles and Shorter was preparing for the Olympic Marathon in Munich. The book is written to help world-class runners, as well as less experienced competitors, to run the best races they can. There are training tips from Shorter, Bill Rodgers, Libbie Hickman, Emil Zatopek, and other famous runners including 75 workouts to create a serious runner's handbook.

Chapter 4: Gymnastics and cheerleading

Chappell, L. R. (2005). *Coaching cheerleading successfully* (2nd edn). Champaign, IL: Human Kinetics

> Linda Ray Chapell shares over 30 years of experience coaching cheerleaders to win special awards and college tryouts.

Gutman, D. (1998). *Gymnastics: the trials, the triumphs, the truth.* New York: Penguin

> Dan Gutman gives biographies of some of the stars of the sport such as Olga Korbut, Nadia Comaneci, Kurt Thomas, Mary Lou Retton, and coach Bela Karolyi. He presents a thought-provoking glimpse of the high price of success in gymnastics as well as taking the reader into the intense world of this gravity-defying sport.

Kogan, K. D. and Vidmar, P. (2000). *Gymnastics.* Morgantown, WV: Sport Psychology Library

> This book is written by Dr Karen Kogan, a former University of California at Los Angeles gymnast and internationally known sports psychologist, and Peter Vidmar, who serves on the executive committee of USA Gymnastics. In 1984, he led the US Olympic men's gymnastics team to its first ever Olympic gold medal while also capturing the gold on the pommel horse and the silver in the All-Around competition. In the book, Olympic gymnasts Shannon Miller, Amanda Borden, Jaycie Phelps, Kerri Strug, and Tim Daggett discuss how important mental skills are in becoming a champion.

Schlegel, E. and Dunn, C. R. (2001). *The gymnastics book: the young performer's guide to gymnastics.* New York: Firefly Books

> This book is basically for beginners, and although it applies to both genders, all of the pictures depict little girls.

Chapter 5: Show jumping

Hale, C. and Fibelkorn, S. P. (2002). *Riding for the blue: a celebration of horse shows.* Irvine, CA: Bow Tie Press

> This book includes how-to approaches, heart-warming stories, and great photography to stimulate anyone interested in further developing in this sport.

Mailer, C. (2005). *Jumping problem solved gridwork: the secret to success.* North Pomfret, VT: Trafalgar Square Publishing

> A comprehensive guide for riders, coaches, and trainers covering both the mental and physical sides to jumping.

Steinkraus, W. (1997). *Reflections on riding and jumping: winning techniques for serious riders*. North Pomfret, VT, Trafalgar Square Publishing

> Bill Steinkraus was the first American to win an Olympic gold medal for show jumping. He was a member of the US Equestrian Team (USET) for 20 years and its riding captain for 16 years. Following his retirement, he served as President and then Chairman of USET. His focus on the mental side of the sport addresses the rider's understanding of the horse and getting the horse mentally correct.

Chapter 6: Football, baseball, and basketball

Brees, D., with Fabry, C. (2010). *Coming back stronger: unleashing the hidden power of adversity*. Carol Stream, IL: Tyndale House

> Drew Brees, the most valuable player in the New Orleans Saints' Super Bowl Championship in February, 2010, talks about rebuilding his own career after a possible vocation-ending shoulder injury, but also helping the City of New Orleans to recover from Hurricane Katrina. This win was the first time the Saints even made it to the championship game. A true inspiration on and off the field, Brees became a symbol of hope to the community. The publishers founded their company to publish religious books, and Brees' faith-based approach to life is evident in his writing.

Jordan, M. (2005). *Driven from within*. New York: Atria Books

> This book, edited by Mark Vancil, presents a mental side of competition as seen through the eyes of Michael Jordan, arguably the best basketball player ever. Jordan was quoted as saying: "The process to me has always been pure. It's about leading and staying true – authentic – to those fundamental values that flowed downstream from my parents and later Coach Dean Smith. Moving through the business world full time, I recognize that the structure of success is no different there than it was on the basketball court. Great companies have a lot in common with great teams. Players who practice hard when no one is paying attention generally play well when everyone is watching. Success at any level can be reverse engineered to reveal the same architecture."

Kriegel, M. (2004). *Namath: a biography*. New York: Penguin

Mark Kriegel does an excellent job of describing Joe Namath's positive approaches to projecting success, including his "guarantee" that the New York Jets, an 18-point underdog, would defeat the heavily favored Baltimore Colts in the 1969 Super Bowl. This was the third year since the championship game between the American Football League (AFL) and National Football League (NFL) had been given this title. The first two were won rather handily by the NFL, and this game was forecast as the most lopsided in the game's short history.

Lombardi, V., Jr. (1991). *What it takes to be #1: Vince Lombardi on leadership*. New York: McGraw-Hill

Vince Lombardi, legendary coach of the Green Bay Packers, is often considered one of the great motivators of men of all times. This book, written by his son, Vince, Jr., relates many stories and quotes about Coach Lombardi and how he molded men. One, for example, had to do with recovery from injury. After the team physician had examined Vince, Jr.'s knee and said it was not anything serious, Coach said to his son: "Stop babying that knee and start running on it," adding: "The Good Lord gave you a body that can withstand just about anything. It is your mind you have to convince."

Marx, J. (2009). *The long snapper: a second chance, a Super Bowl, a lesson for life*. New York: Harper

Jeffrey Marx, author of the bestseller *Season of life*, does a great job of describing the mental anguish experienced by Brian Kinchen when he was called out of retirement by the New England Patriots to be the long snapper in the 2003 Super Bowl. Frank Deford, a *Sports Illustrated* writer, gave the book the following endorsement: "Don't we all long for one last chance? Don't we all dream to do it over again? Anybody who has ever had those pangs will love Jeffrey Marx's beautiful and uplifting story about a guy who had opportunity dropped into his lap. Do yourself a favor and read *The long snapper*."

Payton, S. and Henican, E. (2010). *Home team: coaching the Saints and New Orleans back to life*. New York: New American Library

One of those books that you don't want to put down, it takes the reader through Coach Sean Payton's decision to take the head coaching job of a team that was 3-13 in the season that began just after Hurricane Katrina. He had to move his family to the devastated city, take a chance on an injured quarterback that the San Diego Chargers had given up on, and make his first draft pick Reggie Bush, who didn't want to come to New Orleans. Four years later, the team has gone from one that was displaced from the city – and from a stadium which made the international news and became a symbol of misery and hopelessness because of the horrible conditions there, when it became a shelter of last resort – to 2010 Super Bowl champions. One of the most inspirational aspects of the book is how the players and coaches became a part of rebuilding the city as well as the team, and how the community supported them so devotedly.

Chapter 7: Softball

Solomon, G. and Becker, A. (2004). *Focused on fastpitch.* Champaign, IL: Human Kinetics

> While most of the other softball titles I previewed regarding softball dealt with the mechanics of pitching, hitting, fielding, base running, and so on, this book focused a great deal on the mental side of the sport. It has chapters on "Mentaphysical training: train the mind to improve the body's performance" and "Thinking the game: utilize constructive attitudes and routine to gain the edge." The book aims to help players make the leap from making great plays occasionally to making great plays regularly.
>
> One reviewer says: "The mental side of the game is what raises the bar from good to great on the field and on base paths, and in shutting out distraction in the circle."

Chapter 8: Tennis

Gallwey, W. T. (1974). *The inner game of tennis: the classic guide to the mental side of peak performance* (1st edn). New York: Random House

> The 2008 paperback edition of this book includes an excellent foreword written by Pete Carrol, who through the 2009 football season was Head Coach of the University of Southern California's football team (and from 2010, Head Coach of the Seattle Seahawks in the NFL). He talks about how when introduced to Timothy Gallwey's book years ago, while still an undergraduate, he recognized the obvious benefits

of his techniques with regard to performance in individual sports. Carrol says as he grew more familiar with the benefits of performing with a "quieted mind," he started to cement the principles of trust as characteristics that could also benefit teams.

Gilbert, B. and Jamison, S. (1994). *Winning ugly: mental warfare in tennis – lessons from a master.* New York: Simon & Schuster

Coach Minnis highly recommends this book to anyone who wants to become a serious tennis player, noting that "Brad Gilbert has coached Andre Agassi and Andy Roddick and teaches how to compete and to fight every shot." Agassi has written a chapter for the book and is quoted on the front cover as saying: "*Winning ugly* explains Brad's formula for a winning tennis game. He understands the mental part of tennis better than anyone I have ever met. Brad helped me improve my game and I believe he can help you improve yours."

Greenwald, J. (2007). *The best tennis of your life: 50 mental strategies for fearless performance.* Cincinatti, OH: Betterway Books

Among many other mental aspects discussed, Jeff Greenwald talks about "finding pleasure in pressure." He notes that close matches should be seen as opportunities to challenge yourself, dig deep, and execute your shots regardless of how nervous you feel. When you feel like your back is against the wall, this is the time to reach deeply into your guts and stand tall.

Chapter 9: Volleyball, soccer, shooting, cycling, and rugby

Taylor, J. and Schneider, T. (2005). *The triathlete's guide to mental training.* Boulder, CO: Velo Press

Dr Jim Taylor and Terri Schneider, a former triathlete and considered one of the top female endurance athletes in the world, write about the mental aspects of competition in endurance sports. They note that if two athletes are evenly matched in skill, physical preparation, and equipment, and are pitted against one another head-to-head, the one with the best mental preparation will prevail. They list six psychological factors that might dramatically limit race performance. It is interesting reading for any of the sports covered in this book.

Chapter 10: Sports injuries

Taylor, J., Stone, K. R., Mullen, M. J., Ellenbecker, T., and Walgenbach, A. (2003). *Comprehensive sports injury management: from examination of injury to return to sport.* Austin, TX: Pro-Ed

> Jim Taylor, PhD is internationally recognized for his work in sports psychology and injury rehabilitation. He has been a consultant to the US and Japanese Ski Teams, USA Triathalon, and the United States Tennis Association, and he has worked with injured athletes in a number of professional sports as well as athletes at lower levels. Kevin Stone, MD is an orthopedic surgeon and chairman of the Stone Foundation for Sports Medicine and Arthritis Research. He specializes in sports medicine and is a physician for the US Ski Team as well as various ballet groups, and is a part of the United States Olympic Training Center. The book takes a comprehensive approach to dealing with injured athletes from diagnosis to return to sport.

Taylor, J. and Taylor, S. (1997). *Psychological approaches to sports injury rehabilitation.* Gathersburg, MD: Aspen Publications

> In this book, the authors describe how injuries are inevitable for athletes. At some point, these injuries might take them out of sports for extended times. They note that although most will recover physically, some will suffer psychological effects that will inhibit rehabilitation. For these athletes, working with them to regain self-confidence and motivation, as well as overcoming fear, are often more difficult than their physical recovery.

Chapter 11: Substance abuse

Karch, S. (2009). *Pathology of drug abuse* (4th edn). Boca Raton, FL: Taylor and Francis

> Steven Karch provides a comprehensive review of drugs of abuse and how they have been used by athletes attempting to improve their performance and endurance.

Tramontana, J. (2009). *Hypnotically enhanced treatment for addictions: alcohol abuse, drug abuse, gambling, weight control, and smoking cessation*. Carmarthen, UK: Crown House Publishing

> This book includes scripts, strategies, techniques, and case examples to aid the therapist in designing treatment plans for all addictions, whether working with an athlete or non-athlete.

Wadler, G. I. and Hainline, B. (1989). *Drugs and the athlete.* Philadelphia, PA: F.A. Davis Company

> This book offers a contemporary review of the state of drug abuse in sports up to the late 1980s. Gary Wadler and Brian Hainline give many case examples of athletes who blew opportunities for greatness or had their careers cut short because of drug use.

Movies

Chariots of Fire (1981). This British film tells the fact-based story of two athletes in the 1924 Olympics: Eric Liddell, a devout Scottish Christian, who runs for the glory of God, and Harold Abrahams, an English Jew, who runs to overcome prejudice. Although nominated for seven Academy Awards, this movie was a surprise and upset winner of the Academy Award for best picture in 1981, beating out such box office hits such as *On Golden Pond* and *Raiders of the Lost Ark*. It won three other Oscars as well and it is ranked 19th in the British Film Institute's list of Top 100 British films. It has been suggested that the film's title is a reference to the line, "Bring me my chariot of fire," from the William Blake poem adapted into the hymn "Jerusalem", because the hymn is heard at the end of the film.

Cinderella Man (2005). A biography and drama set during the Great Depression, in which James Braddock (Russell Crowe), a boxer unable to continue to make a constant living through boxing, sets out to do whatever it takes to support his family. Never giving up and determined to succeed and take care of his family, James makes possible what appears to be impossible.

For Love of the Game (2000). A film from the book of the same name is about a supposedly over-the-hill baseball pitcher, played by Kevin Costner, who used a form of self-hypnosis which he refers to as "clear the mechanism" that allows him to block out crowd noise.

Hoosiers (1986). A drama based on the true story of Coach Norman Dale (Gene Hackman) who takes on a high school basketball team in a small town in Indiana. Coach Dale encounters many obstacles and challenges while trying to lead his team to the state finals.

Miracle (2004). A true story of the 1980 US Olympic hockey team, their coach Herb Brooks (Kurt Russell) and the obstacles they faced and had to overcome.

Prefontaine (1997). Written by Steve James and Eugene Carr. Produced by Disney Productions. Based on the life of Steve Prefontaine, an Olympic hopeful who was coached by Bill Bowerman in Oregon. Bowerman was the creator of the Nike running shoe. Prefontaine was considered by many as the best distance runner in the history of American running.

Remember the Titans (2001). A picture from Walt Disney Videos. Many coaches in football and other sports have had their players watch this inspirational movie about the will to win.

Rocky (1976). Rocky Balboa (Sylvester Stallone) gets the chance of a lifetime. A struggling no-name boxer gets the chance to prove his potential and become who he was destined to be.

Without Limits (1998). Written and directed by Robert Towne, and produced by Tom Cruise and Paula Wagner. This is a biographical film about the friendship between running star Steve Prefontaine and his coach Bill Bowerman, who had co-founded Nike, Inc. Billy Crudup plays Prefontaine and Donald Sutherland plays Bowerman. Although the movie did not gross much at the box office, it got excellent reviews and Sutherland won a Golden Globe award for best supporting actor.

References

Allen, R. P. (2004). *Scripts and strategies in hypnotherapy: the complete works.* Carmarthen, UK: Crown House Publishing.

American Psychological Association Division 30 (n.d.). *Hypnosis: what it is and how it can help you feel better.* Washington, DC: Society of Psychological Hypnosis.

Bandler, R. (1982). The healing potential of the human brain. Workshop sponsored by the Institute for Advancement of Human Behavior, Denver, CO.

Bandler, R. and Grinder, J. (1989). *Frogs into princes: neurolinguistic programming.* Moab, UT: Real People Press.

Barber, J. (1990). Examples of preoperative suggestions. In D. C. Hammond (ed.), *Handbook of hypnotic suggestions and metaphors.* New York: W.W. Norton, (p. 98).

Brees, D., with Fabry, C. (2010). *Coming back stronger: unleashing the hidden power of adversity.* Carol Stream, IL: Tyndale House.

Cameron, J. (1993). *The artist's way.* London: Pan Books.

Chappell, L. R. (2005). *Coaching cheerleading successfully* (2nd edn). Champagne, IL: Human Kinetics.

Dyer, W. (2004). *The power of intention.* Carlsbad, CA: Hay House.

Edgette, J. H. and Rowan, T. (2003). *Winning the mind game: using hypnosis in sport psychology.* Carmarthen, UK: Crown House Publishing.

Eimer, B. N. (2002). *Hypnotize yourself out of pain now!* Oakland, CA: New Harbinger.

Ellis, A. E. and Harper, R. A. (1975). *A new guide to rational living.* Englewood Cliffs, NJ: Prentice-Hall.

Erickson, M. H. (1958). Naturalistic techniques of hypnosis. *American Journal of Clinical Hypnosis*, 1, 3–8.

Ewin, D. M. (2008). Ideomotor signaling in the treatment of psychosomatic illness. Workshop sponsored by the New Orleans Society for Clinical Hypnosis, New Orleans, LA.

Ewin, D. M. and Eimer, B. N. (2006). *Ideomotor signals for rapid hypnoanalysis: a how-to manual*. Springfield, IL: Charles Thomas.

Fixx, J. F. (1977). *The complete book of running*. New York: Random House.

Fixx, J. F. (1980). *Jim Fixx's second book of running*. New York: Random House.

Gafner, G. (2008). Communicating with the unconscious. *American Society of Clinical Hypnosis Newsletter* (Spring).

Galloway, J. (2001). *Marathon: you can do it!* Bolinas, CA: Shelter Publications.

Galloway, J. (2002). *Galloway's book on running* (2nd edn). Bolinas, CA: Shelter Publications.

Gallwey, W. T. (1974). *The inner game of tennis: the classic guide to the mental side of peak performance* (1st edn). New York: Random House.

Gallwey, W. T. (1997a). *The inner game of tennis: the classic guide to the mental side of peak performance* (rev. edn). New York: Random House.

Gallwey, W. T. and Kriegel, R. J. (1997b). *Inner skiing* (rev. edn). New York: Random House.

Gallwey, W. T. (1981). *The inner game of golf*. New York: Random House.

Gallwey, W. T. and Kriegel, R. J. (1977). *Inner skiing* (1st edn). New York: Random House.

Garver, R. B. (1990). Chronic pain syndrome. In D. C. Hammond (ed.), *Handbook of hypnotic suggestions and metaphors*. New York: W.W. Norton, pp. 61–62.

Gilbert, B. and Jamison, S. (1994). *Winning ugly: mental warfare in tennis – lessons from a master*. New York: Simon & Schuster.

Ginandes, C., Brooks, P., Sando, W., Jones, C., and Aker, J. (2003). Can medical hypnosis accelerate post-surgical wound healing? Results of a clinical trial. *American Journal of Clinical Hypnosis*, 45, 333–351.

Greenwald, J. (2007). *The best tennis of your life: 50 mental strategies for fearless performance*. Cincinnati, OH: Betterway Books.

Gregg, D. M. (1973). Analeptic circle. In American Society of Clinical Hypnosis, *A syllabus on hypnosis and a handbook of therapeutic suggestions*. Des Plaines, IL: ASCH Education and Research Foundation, pp. 25–26.

Gutman, D. (1998). *Gymnastics: the trials, the triumphs, the truth.* New York: Penguin.

Hale, C. and Fibelkorn, S. P. (2002). *Riding for the blue: a celebration of horse shows.* Irvine, CA: Bow Tie Press.

Hammond, D. C. (ed.) (1990). *Handbook of hypnotic suggestions and metaphors.* New York: W.W. Norton.

Hartland, J. (1966). *Medical and dental hypnosis.* London: Tindale and Cassell.

Havens, R. and Walters, C. (1989). *Hypnotherapy scripts: a neo-Ericksonian approach to persuasive healing.* New York: Brunner/Mazel.

Higdon, H. (1997). *How to train: the best programs, workouts, and schedules for runners of all ages.* Emmaus, PN: Rodale Press.

Hilgard, E. R. and Hilgard, J. R. (1994). *Hypnosis in the relief of pain.* Levittown, PA: Brunner/Mazel.

Hill, N. (1938). *Think and grow rich.* Meriden, CT: The Ralston Society.

Hodenfield, C. (2009). Mental edge. *Delta Sky Magazine* (August), pp. 76–86.

Johnson, W. R. (1961). Body movement awareness in the nonhypnotic and hypnotic states. *Research Quarterly*, 32, 263–264.

Jordan, M. (2005). *Driven from within.* New York: Atria Books.

Karch, S. (2009). *Pathology of drug abuse* (4th edn). Boca Raton, FL: Taylor and Francis.

King, B. J. and Brennan, C. (2008). *Pressure is a privilege: lessons I've learned from life and the battle of the sexes.* New York: Life Time Media.

King, P. (1996). Five questions. *Sports Illustrated* (July 15), pp. 74–79.

Kogan, K. D. and Vidmar, P. (2000). *Gymnastics.* Morgantown, WV: Sport Psychology Library.

Kriegel, M. (2004). *Namath: a biography.* New York: Penguin.

Kroger, W. S. and Fezler, W. D. (1976). *Hypnosis and behavior modification: imagery conditioning.* Philadelphia, PA: J.B. Lippincott Company.

Lesyk, J. L. (1998). *Developing sport psychology within your clinical practice: a practical guide for mental health professionals.* San Francisco, CA: Jossey-Bass.

Liggett, D. R. (2000). *Sport hypnosis*. Champaign, IL: Human Kinetics.

Loehr, J. (1995). *The new toughness training for sports: mental, emotional, physical conditioning from one of the world's premier sports psychologists*. New York: Penguin.

Loehr, J. (2010). Building a career in sport psychology: my insights, my struggles, my story. Keynote lecture delivered at the 25th Annual Conference of the Association of Applied Sport Psychology, Providence, RI.

Lombardi, V., Jr. (1991). *What it takes to be #1: Vince Lombardi on leadership*. New York: McGraw-Hill.

Look, C. (1997). Cell by cell: accessing your body's natural healing abilities. *Hypnotherapy Today* (July), pp. 1–2.

McDougall, C. (2009). *Born to run: a hidden tribe, superathletes, and the greatest race the world has never seen*. New York: Knopf.

Mack, G. and Casstevens, D. (2001). *Mind gym: an athlete's guide to inner excellence*. Chicago, IL: Contemporary Books.

Mailer, C. (2005). *Jumping problem solved gridwork: the secret to success*. North Pomfret, VT: Trafalgar Square Publishing.

Marshall, M. (2001). Mike Marshall on the mental side of pitching. *Coach and Athletic Director* (May 1). Available at www.allbusiness.com/ sector-61-educational-services/543942-1.html.

Marx, J. (2003). *Season of life: a football star, a boy, a journey to manhood*. New York: Simon & Schuster.

Marx, J. (2009). *The long snapper: a second chance, a Super Bowl, a lesson for life*. New York: HarperCollins.

Meichenbaum, D. (1977). *Cognitive-behavior modification*. New York: Plenum Press.

Miller, S. D. and Berg, I. K. (1995). *The miracle method: a radically new approach to problem drinking*. New York: Norton.

Morgan, W. P. (2002). Hypnosis in sport and exercise psychology. In J. L. Van Raalte and B. W. Brewer (eds), *Exploring sport and exercise psychology*. Washington, DC: American Psychological Association, pp. 151–181.

Payton, S. and Henican, E. (2010). *Home team: coaching the Saints and New Orleans back to life*. New York: New American Library.

Phillips, M. (2007). *Reversing chronic pain: a 10-point all-natural plan for lasting relief*. Berkeley, CA: North Atlantic Books.

Pulos, L. (1990). *Beyond hypnosis*. Vancouver: Omega Press.

Pulos, L. and Smith, M. (1998). Sports medicine. Workshop presented at the 40th Annual Scientific Meeting of the American Society of Clinical Hypnosis, Fort Worth, TX.

Pratt, G. J. and Korn, E. R. (1996).Using hypnosis to enhance athletic performance. In B. Zilbergeld, M. G. Edelstein, and D. L. Araoz (eds), *Hypnosis: questions and answers*. New York: W.W. Norton, pp. 337–342.

Robbins, A. (1986). *Unlimited power* (audiobook). New York: Simon & Schuster.

Rotella, R. (1995). *Golf is not a game of perfect*. New York: Simon & Schuster.

Rotella, R. (1996). *Golf is a game of confidence*. New York: Simon & Schuster.

Rotella, R. (2004). *The golfer's mind*. New York: Simon & Schuster.

Rossi, E. L. and Cheek, D. B. (1988). *Mind-body therapy: methods of ideodynamic healing in hypnosis*. New York: W.W. Norton.

Sandrock, M. (2001). *Running tough*. Champaign, IL. Human Kinetics.

Saunders, T. (2005). *Golf: lower your score with mental training*. Carmarthen, UK: Crown House Publishing.

Schlegel, E. and Dunn, C. R. (2001). *The gymnastics book: the young performer's guide to gymnastics*. New York: Firefly Books.

Schwartz, D. (2008). Brains and brawn. *Monitor on Psychology*, 39(7), 54–56.

Selye, H. (1956). *The stress of life*. New York: McGraw-Hill.

Shipnuck, A. (2009). Last man standing. *Sports Illustrated* (April 20), pp. 30–34.

Smith, M. (2009). Sports hypnosis. Workshop presented at the 51st Annual Scientific Meeting of the American Society of Clinical Hypnosis, Boston, MA.

Solomon, G. and Becker, A. (2004). *Focused on fastpitch*. Champaign, IL: Human Kinetics.

Steinkraus, W. (1997). *Reflections on riding and jumping: winning techniques for serious riders*. North Pomfret, VT: Trafalgar Square Publishing.

Sylvester, S. M. (1990). Preparation for surgery. In D. C. Hammond (ed.), *Handbook of hypnotic suggestions and metaphors*. New York: W.W. Norton, pp. 98–101.

Taylor, J. and Schneider, T. (2005). *The triathlete's guide to mental training*. Boulder, CO: VeloPress.

Taylor, J., Stone, K. R., Mullin, M. J., Ellenbecker, T., and Walgenbach, A. (2003). *Comprehensive sports injury management: from examination of injury to return to sport*. Austin, TX: Pro-Ed.

Taylor, J. and Taylor, S. (1997). *Psychological approaches to sports injury rehabilitation*. Gathersburg, MD: Aspen Publications.

Thompson, R. A. and Sherman, R. T. (1993). *Helping athletes with eating disorders: a user's guide*. Champaign, IL: Human Kinetics.

Tramontana, J. (1983). Subject bias as a significant factor in hypnotic inductions with child clients. *Hypnotherapy Today* (December), p. 1.

Tramontana, J. (2005). Hypnotherapy and hypnosis as an adjunctive technique in psychotherapy. Continuing education unit seminar presented at the Veterans Administration Hospital, Gulfport, MS.

Tramontana, J. (2008a). HEAT: hypnotically enhanced addictions treatment: an overview. Workshop presented at the 58th Annual Convention of the Mississippi Psychological Association; Tunica, MS.

Tramontana, J. (2008b). Successful blepharoplasty with self-hypnosis, a spousal "coach," and only local anesthesia: a case report. *Psychological Hypnosis: A Bulletin of APA Division 30*, 17(3), 4–7.

Tramontana, J. (2009a). *Hypnotically enhanced treatment for addictions: alcohol abuse, drug abuse, gambling, weight control, and smoking cessation*. Carmarthen, UK: Crown House Publishing.

Tramontana, J. (2009b). Hypnotically enhanced treatment of addictions: strategies, techniques, scripts. Workshop presented at the 51st Annual Scientific Meeting of the American Society of Clinical Hypnosis, Boston, MA.

Tramontana, J. (2009c). Hypnotically enhanced addictions treatment (HEAT): strategies, techniques, script, and case examples. Workshop presented at the 55th Annual Convention of the Louisiana Psychological Association, Baton Rouge, LA.

Van Raalte, J. L. and Brewer, B. W. (eds) (2002). *Exploring sport and exercise psychology*. Washington, DC: American Psychological Association.

Wadler, G. I. and Hainline, B. (1989). *Drugs and the athlete*. Philadelphia, PA: F.A. Davis Company.

Wark, D. M. (2008). From the president's desk. *American Society of Clinical Hypnosis Newsletter* (Fall), p. 1.

Wark, D. M. (2009). Alert hypnosis: using hypnotic phenomena with your eyes wide open. Workshop sponsored by the New Orleans Society for Clinical Hypnosis, New Orleans, LA.

Wester, W. C. (2007). *Question and answers about clinical hypnosis*. Columbus, OH: Ohio Psychology Publications.

Williams, J. M. and Leffingwell, T. R. (2002). Cognitive strategies in sport and exercise psychology. In J. L. Van Raalte and B. W. Brewer (eds), *Exploring sport and exercise psychology*. Washington, DC: American Psychological Association, pp. 75–98.

Woodcock, C., Sharp, L. A., Holland, M. J. G., Fisher, B., Duda, J. and Cummins, J. (2010). An action research approach to mental skills training: experience, evaluation and evolution. Workshop presented at the 25th Annual Conference of the Association of Applied Sports Psychology, Porvidence, RI.

Index